Textbook of Mental Health and Hygiene

G.D. Gururani

AKANSHA PUBLISHING HOUSE
NEW DELHI • GUWAHATI • VISAKHAPATNAM

AKANSHA PUBLISHING HOUSE
4649-B/21, Ansari Road
Darya Ganj, New Delhi - 110 002
Ph.: 23263193 / 9811582579 / 09435116718
Fax: 011-23263193
Email: ektabooks@yahoo.com
www.akanshapublishinghouse.com

Textbook of Mental Health and Hygiene

First Published 2006
First Reprint 2006
Second Reprint 2009
Third Reprint 2012
Fourth Reprint 2018
Fifth Reprint 2026

PRINTED IN INDIA

Published by Akansha Publishing House, New Delhi and Printed at Harmain Offset, Delhi.

Contents

Preface

> As tools become rusty, so does the mind; a garden uncared for soon becomes smothered in weeds; a talent neglected withers and dies.
>
> —*Ethel R. Page*

Mental hygiene presents the ideal conditions for growth and development of sound mental health. It is a prerequisite for teachers and pupil—both. A teacher, while has to maintain sound mental health himself/herself on the one hand, has the responsibility to keep the vigil on the mental health status of students on the other. Hence the need of the study of mental health and mental hygiene.

There are many factors responsible for mental illness of one sort of another which ultimately hampers the teaching-learning process as well as the personality development of the concerned person. An understanding of these factors may lead us to overcome the illness. There are three groups of mental disorders: (1) Psychoses; (2) Neuroses, personality disorders and other non-psychotic disorders; and (3) Mental impairment.

Here we have collated eleven relevant articles which X-ray the factors responsible for mental hygiene and mental healthin pros and cons. We have drawn upon experiences (works) of many distinguished psychologists and psychiatrist so that the book could be helpful with authoritative information.

The main themes included herein are—Fundamentals of Mental Health; Mental Health of Children; Adults and Mental Health; Intelligence and Mental Processes; Mental Health

Services: Organisation; Mental Retardation in India; Mental Hygiene and Role of Councellor; Forgetting; Mental Hygiene and Memory; Infants' Movements; Suggestions etc. An elaborate bibliography and Glossary of terms at the end of the book will enhance its utility.

While compiling the material we have to consult many libraries. We owe a deep sense of gratitude to different librarians. Since the information contained herein is drawn from different sources—all secondary, we are deeply beholden to all those whose works are cited or substantially made use of. Friends and family members deserve all appreciation for their constant moral support, inspiration and all possible assistance.

Finally we are thankful to our publishers for materializing our efforts in nice way.

Suggestion and constructive criticism from all quarters are welcome which will make the subsequent edition of the book more useful and informative.

—Editor

1

Fundamentals of Mental Health

> Men become bad and guilty because they speak and act without foreseeing the results of their words and their deeds.
>
> —*Franz Kafka*

Modern integrative neuroscience offers a means of linking research on broad "systems level" aspects of brain function with the remarkably detailed tools and findings of molecular biology. All of human behavior is mediated by the brain. Consider, for example, a memory that most people have from childhood—that of learning to ride a bicycle with the help of a parent or friend. The fear of falling, the anxiety of lack of control, the reassurances of a loved one, and the final liberating experience of mastery and a newly extended universe create an unforgettable combination. For some, the memories are not good ones: falling and being chased by dogs have left marks of anxiety and fear that may last a lifetime. Science is revealing how the skill learning, emotional overtones, and memories of such experiences are put together physically in the brain. The brain and mind are two sides of the same coin. Mind is not possible without the remarkable physical complexity that is built into the brain, but, in addition, the physical complexity of the brain is useless without the sculpting that environment, experience, and thought itself provides. Thus the brain is now known to be physically shaped by contributions from our genes and our experience, working together. This strengthens the view that mental disorders are both caused and can be treated by biological and experiential processes, working together. This understanding has emerged from the breathtaking progress in modern neuroscience that has begun to integrate knowledge from biological and behavioral sciences.

An overview of mental illness follows the section on modern integrative brain science. The section highlights topics including symptoms, diagnosis, epidemiology (i.e., research having to do with the distribution and determinants of mental disorders in population groups, including various racial and ethnic minority groups), and cost, all of which are discussed in greater and more pointed detail in the chapters that follow. Etiology is the study of the origins and causes of disease, and that section reviews research that is seeking to define, with ever greater precision, the causes of mental disorders. As will be seen, etiology research examines fundamental biological, behavioral, and sociocultural processes, as well as a necessarily broad array of life events. The section on development of temperament reveals how mental health science has attempted over much of the past century to understand how biological, psychological, and sociocultural factors meld in health as well as in illness. The chapter then reviews research approaches to the prevention and treatment of mental disorders and provides an overview of mental health services and their delivery. Final sections cover the growing influence on the mental health field of the need for attention to cultural diversity, the importance of the consumer movement, and new optimism about recovery from mental illness—that is, the possibility of recovering one's life.

Structural Complexity of the Brain

As befits the organ of the mind, the human brain is the most complex structure ever investigated by our science. The brain contains approximately 100 billion nerve cells, or neurons, and many more supporting cells, or ganglia. In and of themselves, the number of cells in this 3-pound organ reveal little of its complexity. Yet most organs in the body are composed of only a handful of cell types; the brain, in contrast, has literally thousands of different kinds of neurons, each distinct in terms of its chemistry, shape, and connections (Figure 1 depicts the structural variety of neurons). To illustrate, one careful, recent investigation of a kind of interneuron that is a small local circuit neuron in the retina, called the amacrine cell, found no less than 23 identifiable types.

But this is only the beginning of the brain's complexity.

The workings of the brain depend on the ability of nerve cells to communicate with each other. Communication occurs at small, specialized structures called synapses. The synapse typically has two parts. One is a specialized presynaptic structure on a terminal portion of the sending neuron that contains packets of signaling chemicals, or neurotransmitters. The second is a postsynaptic structure on the dendrites of the receiving neuron that has receptors for the neurotransmitter molecules.

The typical neuron has a cell body, which contains the genetic material, and much of the cell's energy-producing machinery. Emanating from the cell body are dendrites, branches that are the most important receptive surface of the cell for communication. The dendrites of neurons can assume a great many shapes and sizes, all relevant to the way in which incoming messages are processed. The output of neurons is carried along what is usually a single branch called the axon. It is down this part of the neuron that signals are transmitted out to the next neuron. At its end, the axon may branch into many terminals.

The usual form of communication involves electrical signals that travel within neurons, giving rise to chemical signals that diffuse, or cross, synapses, which in turn give rise to new electrical signals in the postsynaptic neuron.

Each neuron, on average, makes more than 1,000 synaptic connections with other neurons. One type of cell—a Purkinje cell—may make between 100,000 and 200,000 connections with other neurons. In aggregate, there may be between 100 trillion and a quadrillion synapses in the brain. These synapses are far from random. Within each region of the brain, there is an exquisite architecture consisting of layers and other anatomic substructures in which synaptic connections are formed. Ultimately, the pattern of synaptic connections gives rise to what are called circuits in the brain. At the integrative level, large- and small-scale circuits are the substrates of behavior and of mental life. One of the most awe-inspiring mysteries of brain science is how neuronal activity within circuits gives rise to behavior and, even, consciousness.

The complexity of the brain is such that a single neuron may be part of more than one circuit. The organization of circuits in the brain reveals that the brain is a massively parallel, distributed information processor. For example, the circuits involved in vision receive information from the retina. After initial processing, these circuits analyze information into different streams, so that there is one stream of information describing what the visual object is, and another stream is concerned with where the object is in space. The information stream having to do with the identity of the object is actually broken down into several more refined parallel streams. One, for example, analyzes shape while another analyzes color. Ultimately, the visual world is resynthesized with information about the tactile world, and the auditory world, with information from memory, and with emotional coloration. The massively parallel design is a great pattern recognizer and very tolerant of failure in individual elements. This is why a brain of neurons is still a better and longer-lasting information processor than a computer.

The specific connectivity of circuits is, to some degree, stereotyped, or set in expected patterns within the brain, leading to the notion that certain places in the brain are specialized for certain functions (Figure 3). Thus, the cerebral cortex, the mantle of neurons with its enormous surface area increased by outpouchings, called gyri, and indentations, called sulci, can be functionally subdivided. The back portion of the cerebral cortex (i.e., the occipital lobe), for example, is involved in the initial stages of visual processing. Just behind the central sulcus is the part of the cerebral cortex involved in the processing of tactile information (i.e., parietal lobe). Just in front of the central sulcus is a part of the cerebral cortex involved in motor behavior (frontal lobe). In the front of the brain is a region called the prefrontal cortex, which is involved with some of the highest integrated functions of the human being, including the ability to plan and to integrate cognitive and emotional streams of information.

Beneath the cortex are enormous numbers of axons sheathed in the insulating substance, myelin. This subcortical "white matter," so named because of its appearance on freshly cut brain sections, surrounds deep aggregations of neurons, or "gray matter," which, like the cortex, appears gray because of the presence of neuronal cell bodies. It is within this gray matter that the brain processes information. The white matter is akin to wiring that conveys information from one region to another. Gray matter regions include the basal ganglia, the part of the brain that is involved in the initiation of motion and thus profoundly affected in Parkinson's disease, but that is also involved in the integration of motivational states and, thus, a substrate of addictive disorders. Other important gray matter structures in the brain include the amygdala and the hippocampus. The amygdala is involved in the assignment of emotional meaning to events and objects, and it appears to play a special role in aversive, or negative, emotions such as fear. The hippocampus includes, among its many functions, responsibility for initially encoding and consolidating explicit or episodic memories of persons, places, and things.

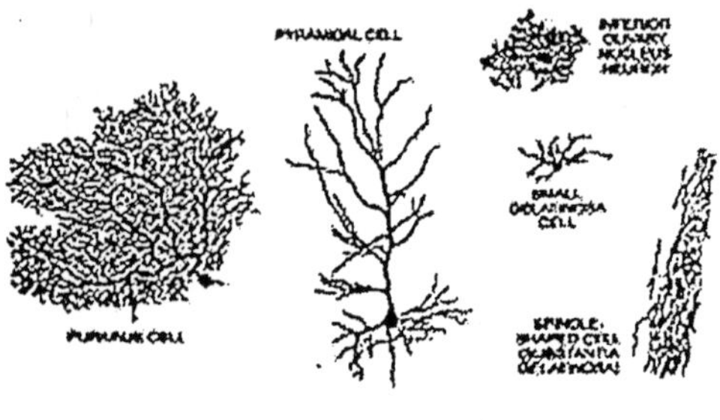

Figure 1. Structural variety of neurons

Source: Fischbach, 1992, p. 53.

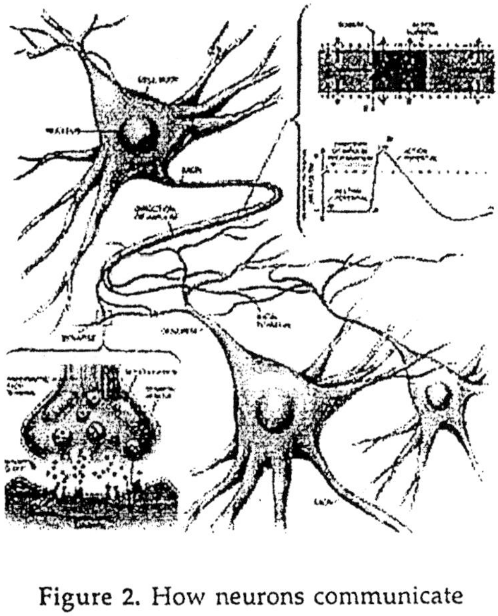

Figure 2. How neurons communicate

Source: Fischbach, 1992, p. 52.

In summary, the organization of the brain at the cellular level involves many thousands of distinct kinds of neurons. At a higher integrative level, these neurons form circuits for information processing determined by their patterns of synaptic connections. The organization of these parallel distributed circuits results in the specialization of different geographic regions of the brain for different functions. It is important to state at this point, however, that, especially in younger individuals, damage to a particular brain region may yield adaptations that permit circuits spared the damage and, therefore, other regions of the brain, to pick up some of the functions that would otherwise have been lost.

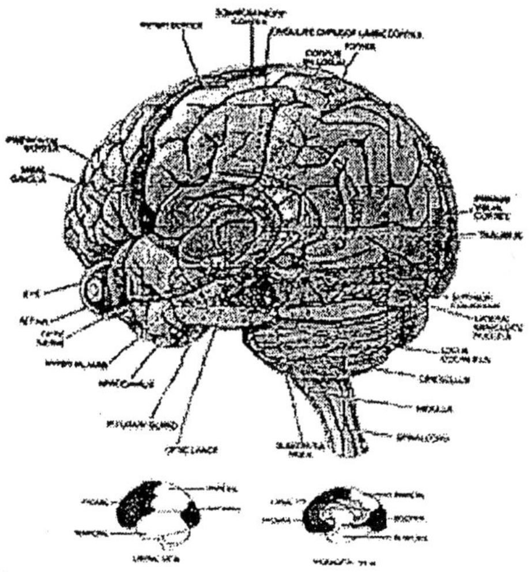

Figure 3. The brain: Organ of the mind

Source: Fischbach, 1992, p. 51.

Neurochemical Complexity of the Brain

Superimposed on this breathtaking structural complexity is the chemical complexity of the brain. As described above, electrical signals within neurons are converted at synapses into chemical signals which then elicit electrical signals on the other side of the synapse. These chemical signals are molecules called neurotransmitters. There are two major kinds of molecules that serve the function of neurotransmitters: small molecules, some quite well known, with names such as dopamine, serotonin, or norepinephrine, and larger molecules, which are essentially protein chains, called peptides.

These include the endogenous opiates, Substance P, and corticotropin releasing factor (CRF), among others. All told, there appear to be more than 100 different neurotransmitters in the brain.

A neurotransmitter can elicit a biological effect in the postsynaptic neuron by binding to a protein called a neurotransmitter receptor. Its job is to pass the information contained in the neurotransmitter message from the synapse to the inside of the receiving cell. It appears that almost every known neurotransmitter has more than one different kind of receptor that can confer rather different signals on the receiving neuron. Dopamine has 5 known neurotransmitter receptors; serotonin has at least 14.

Although there are many kinds of receptors with many different signaling functions, we can divide most neurotransmitter receptors into two general classes. One class of neurotransmitter receptor is called a ligand-gated channel, where "ligand" simply means a molecule (i.e., a neurotransmitter) that binds to a receptor. When neurotransmitters interact with this kind of receptor, a pore within the receptor molecule itself is opened and positive or negative charges enter the cell. The entry of positive charge may activate additional ion channels that allow more positive charge to enter. At a certain threshold, this causes a cell to fire an action potential—an electrical event that leads ultimately to the release of neurotransmitter. By definition, therefore, receptors that admit positive charge are excitatory neurotransmitter receptors. The classic excitatory neurotransmitter receptors in the brain utilize the excitatory amino acids glutamate and, to a lesser degree, aspartate as neurotransmitters. Conversely, inhibitory neurotransmitters act by permitting negative charges into the cell, taking the cell farther away from firing. The classic inhibitory neurotransmitters in the brain are the amino acids gamma amino butyric acid, or GABA, and, to a lesser degree, glycine.

Most of the other neurotransmitters in the brain, such as dopamine, serotonin, and norepinephrine, and all of the many neuropeptides constitute the second major class. These are neither precisely excitatory nor inhibitory but rather act to produce complex biochemical changes in the receiving cell. Their receptors do not contain intrinsic ion pores but rather interact with signaling proteins, called"G proteins" found inside the cell membrane. These receptors thus are called G protein-linked receptors. The details are less important than understanding the general scheme. Stimulation of G protein-linked receptors alters the way in which receiving neurons can process subsequent signals from glutamate or GABA. To use a metaphor of a musical instrument, if glutamate, the excitatory neurotransmitter, is puffing wind into a flute or clarinet, it is the modulatory neurotransmitters such as dopamine or serotonin that might be seen as playing the keys and, thus, altering the melody via G protein-linked receptors.

The architecture of these systems drives home this point. The precise brain circuits that carry specific information about the world and that are involved in precise point-to-point communication within the brain use excitatory or inhibitory neurotransmission. Examples of such circuits, which are massively parallel, can be found in the visual and auditory cortex. Overlying this pattern of precise, rapid (timing in the range of milliseconds) neurotransmission are the modulatory systems in the brain that use norepinephrine, serotonin, and dopamine. In each case, the neurotransmitter in question is made by a very small number of nerve cells clustered in a limited number of areas in the brain. Of the hundred billion neurons in the brain, only about 500,000, for example, make dopamine—that is, for every 200,000 cells in the brain, only one makes dopamine. Even fewer make norepinephrine. The cell bodies of the dopamine neurons are clustered in a few brain regions, most importantly, regions deep in the brain, in the *midbrain,* called the *substantia nigra,* and the *ventral tegmental area.* Norepinephrine neurons are made in the nucleus *locus coeruleus* even farther down in the brain stem in a structure called the *pons.* Serotonin is made by a somewhat larger number of nuclei but, still, not by many cells. Nuclei called the *raphe nuclei* spread along the brain stem. While each of these neurotransmitters is made by a small number of neurons with clustered cell bodies, each sends its axons branching throughout the brain, so that in each case a very small number of neurons, which largely appear to fire in unison when excited, influence almost the entire brain. This is not the picture of systems that are communicating precise bits of information about the world but rather are intrinsic modulatory systems that act via other G protein-linked receptors to alter the overall responsiveness of the brain. These neurotransmitters are responsible for brain states such as degree of arousal, ability to pay attention, and for putting emotional color or significance on top of cold cognitive information provided by precise glutaminergic circuits. It is no wonder that these modulatory neurotransmitters and their receptors are critical targets of medications used to treat mental disorders—for example, the antidepressant and antipsychotic drugs—and also are the targets of drugs of abuse.

Plasticity Complexity of the Brain

The preceding paragraphs have illustrated the chemical and anatomic structure of the brain and, in so doing, provided some picture of its complexity as well as some picture of its function. The crowning complexity of the brain, however, is that it is not static. The brain is always changing. People learn so much and have so many distinct types of memory: conscious, episodic memory of the sort that is encoded initially in the hippocampus; memory of motor programs or procedures that are encoded in the striatum; emotional memories that can initiate physiologic and behaviorally adaptive repertoires encoded, for example, in the amygdala; and many other kinds. Every time a person learns something new, whether it is conscious or unconscious, that experience alters the structure of the brain. Thus, neurotransmission in itself not only contains current information but alters subsequent neurotransmission if it occurs with the right intensity and the right pattern. Experience that is salient enough to cause memory creates new synaptic connections, prunes away old ones, and strengthens or weakens existing ones. Similarly, experiences as diverse as stress, substance abuse, or disease can kill neurons, and current data suggest that new neurons continue to develop even in adult brains, where they help to incorporate new memories. The end result is that information is now routed over an altered circuit. Many of these changes are long-lived, even permanent. It is in this way that a person can look back 10 or 20 or 50 years and remember family, a home or school room, or friends. The general theme is that to really understand the kind of memory—indeed, any brain function—one must think at least at two levels: one, the level of molecular and cellular alterations that are responsible for remodeling synapses, and, two, the level of information content and behavior which circuits and synapses serve.

To conclude, scientists are truly beginning to learn about the structure and function of the brain. Its awe-inspiring complexity is fully consistent with the fact that it supports all behavior and mental life. Implied in the foregoing, is the fact that brains are built not only by genes—and again, it is the lion's share of the 80,000 or so human genes that are involved in building a structure so complex as the brain. Genes are not by themselves the whole story. Brains are built and changed through life through the interaction of genes with environment, including experience. It is true that a set of genes might create repetitive multiples of one type of unit, yet the brain appears far more complex than that. It stands to reason that if 50,000 or 60,000 genes are involved in building a brain that may have 100 trillion or a quadrillion synapses, additional information is needed, and that information comes from the environment. It is this fundamental realization that is beginning to permit an understanding of how treatment of mental disorders works—whether in the form of a somatic intervention such as a medication, or a psychological "talk" therapy—by actually changing the brain.

There are many exciting developments in brain science. Of great relevance to the study of mental function and mental illness is the ability to image the activity of the living human brain with technologies developed in recent decades, such as positron emission tomography scanning or functional magnetic resonance imaging. Such approaches can exploit surrogates of neuronal firing such as blood flow and blood oxygenation to provide maps of activity. As science learns more about brain circuitry and learns more from cognitive and affective neuroscience about how to activate and examine the function of particular brain circuits, differences between health and illness in the function of particular circuits certainly will become evident. We will be able to see the action of psychotropic drugs and, perhaps most exciting, we will be able to see the impact of that special kind of learning called psychotherapy, which works after all because it works on the brain.

Different brain chemicals, brain receptors, and brain structures will come up in the discussion of particular illnesses throughout this document. This section is meant to provide a panoramic, not a detailed, introduction and also to provide certain overarching lessons. When something is referred to as biological or brain-based, that is not shorthand for saying it is genetic and, thus, predetermined; similarly, references to "psychological" or even "social" phenomena do not exclude biological processes. The brain is the great integrator, bringing together genes and environment. The study of the brain requires reducing problems initially to bite-sized bits that will allow investigators to learn something, but ultimately, the agenda of neuroscience is not reductionist; the goal is to understand behavior, not to put blinders on and try to explain it away. As the foregoing discussion illustrates, the brain also is complex. Thus, having a disease that affects one or even many critical circuits does not overthrow, except in extreme cases, such as advanced Alzheimer's disease, all aspects of a person.

Early biological models of the mind seem impoverished and deterministic—for example, models that held that "levels" of a neurotransmitter such as serotonin in the brain were the principal influence on whether one was depressed or aggressive. Neuroscience is far beyond that now, working to integrate information coming "bottom-up" from genes and molecules and cells, with information flowing "top-down" from interactions with the environment and experience to the internal workings of the mind and its neuronal circuits. Ultimately, however, the goal is not only human self-understanding. In knowing eventually precisely what goes wrong in what circuits and what synapses and with what chemical signals, the hope is to develop treatments with greater effectiveness and with fewer side effects. Indeed, as the following chapters indicate, the hope is for cures and ultimately for prevention.

REVIEW QUESTIONS

1. Explain the chief characteristics of mental health among adults.
2. What are anxiety disorders prevalent among adults?
3. What is mood disorder?
4. Write a note on mental health in adulthood.

2

Mental Health of Children

> Those who follow the banners of reason are like the well-disciplined battalions which, wearing a more sober uniform and making a less dazzling show than the light troops commanded by imagination, enjoy more safety, and even more honour, in conflicts of human life.
>
> —*Sir Walter Scott*

Childhood and adolescence spanning about 20 years, are marked by dramatic changes in physical, cognitive, and social-emotional skills and capacities. Mental health in childhood and adolescence is defined by the achievement of expected developmental cognitive, social, and emotional milestones and by secure attachments, satisfying social relationships, and effective coping skills. Mentally healthy children and adolescents enjoy a positive quality of life; function well at home, in school, and in their communities; and are free of disabling symptoms of psychopathology (Hoagwood et al., 1996).

The basic principles for understanding health and illness apply to children and adolescents, but it is important to underscore the often heard admonition that"children are not little adults." Even more than is true for adults, children must be seen in the context of their social environments, that is, family, peer group, and their larger physical and cultural surroundings. Childhood mental health is expressed in this context, as children proceed through development.

Development, characterized by periods of transition and reorganization, is the focus of much research on children and adolescents. Studies focus on normal and abnormal development, trying to understand and predict the forces that will keep children and adolescents mentally healthy and maintain them on course to become mentally healthy adults. These studies ask what places some at risk for mental illness and what protects some but not others, despite exposure to the same risk factors.

In addition to studies of normal development and of risk factors, much additional research focuses on mental illness in childhood and adolescence and what can be done to prevent or treat it. The science is challenging because of the ongoing process of development. The normally developing child hardly stays the same long enough to make stable measurements. Adult criteria for illness can be difficult to apply to children and adolescents, when the signs and symptoms of mental disorders are often also the characteristics of normal development. For example, a temper tantrum could be an expected behavior in a young child but not in an adult. At some point, however, it becomes clearer that certain symptoms and behaviors cause great distress and may lead to dysfunction of children, their family, and others in their social environment. At these points, it is helpful to consider serious deviations from expected cognitive, social, and emotional development as"mental disorders." Specific treatments and services are available for children and adolescents with such mental disorders, but one cannot forget that these disorders emerge in the context of an ongoing developmental process and shifting relationships within the family and community. These developmental factors must be carefully addressed, if one is to maximize the healthy development of children with mental disorders, promote remediation of associated impairments, and enhance their adult outcomes.

The developmental perspective helps us understand how estimated prevalence rates for mental disorders in children and adolescents vary as a function of the degree of impairment that the child experiences in association with specific symptom patterns. For example, the MECA Study (Methodology for Epidemiology of Mental Disorders in Children and Adolescents) estimated that almost 21 percent of U.S. children ages 9 to 17 had a diagnosable mental or addictive disorder associated with at least minimum impairment. When diagnostic criteria required the presence of *significant* functional impairment, estimates dropped to 11 percent. This estimate translates into a total of 4 million youth who suffer from a major mental illness that results in significant impairments at home, at school, and with peers. Finally, when *extreme* functional impairment is the criterion, the estimates dropped to 5 percent.

Given the process of development, it is not surprising that these disorders in some youth are known to wax and wane, such that some afflicted children improve as development unfolds, perhaps as a result of healthy influences impinging on them. Similarly, other youth, formerly only "at risk," may develop full-blown forms of disorder, as severe and devastating in their impact on the youth and his or her family as are the analogous conditions that affect adults. Characterizing such disorders as relatively unchangeable underestimates the potential beneficial influences that can redirect a child whose development has gone awry. Likewise, characterizing children with mental disorders as "only" the victims of negative environmental influences that might be fixed if societal factors were just changed runs the risk of underestimating the severity of these conditions and the need for focused, intensive clinical interventions for suffering children and adolescents. Thus, the science of mental health in childhood and adolescence is a complex mix of the study of development and the study of discrete conditions or disorders. Both perspectives are useful. Each alone has its limitations, but together they constitute a more fully informed approach that spans mental health and illness *and* allows one to design developmentally informed strategies for prevention and treatment.

Normal Development

Development is the lifelong process of growth, maturation, and change that unfolds at the fastest pace during childhood and adolescence. An appreciation of normal development is crucial to understanding mental health in children and adolescents and the risks they face in maintaining mental health. Distortions in the process of development may lead to mental disorders. This section deals with the normal development of understanding (cognitive development) in young children and the development of social relationships and temperament.

Theories of Development

Historically, the changes that take place in a child's psyche between birth and adulthood were largely ignored. Child development first became a subject of serious inquiry at the beginning of this century but was mostly viewed from the perspective of mental disorders and from the cultural mainstream of Europe and white America. Some of the"grand theories" of child development, such as that propounded by Sigmund Freud, grew out of this focus, and they unquestionably drew attention to the importance of child development in laying the foundation for adult mental health. Even those theories that resulted from the observation of healthy children, such as Piaget's theory of cognitive development, paid little attention to the relationship between the development of the"inner self" and the environment into which the individual was placed. In contrast, the interaction of an individual with the environment was central to the school of thought known as behaviorism.

Theories of normal development, are presented briefly below, because they form the basis of many current approaches to understanding and treating mental illness and mental health problems in children and adults. These theories have not achieved the broader objective of explaining how children grow into healthy adults. More study and perhaps new theories will be needed to improve our ability to guide healthy child-rearing with scientific evidence.

Development Viewed as a Series of Stages

Freud and the psychoanalyst Erik Erikson proposed a series of stages of development reflecting the attainment of biological objectives. The stages are expressed in terms of functioning as an individual and with others—within the family and the broader social environment (particularly in Erikson's theories). Although criticized as unscientific and relevant primarily to the era and culture in which they were conceived, these theories introduced the importance of thinking developmentally, that is, of considering the ever-changing physical and psychological capacities and tasks faced by people as they age. They emphasized the concept of "maturation" and moving through the stages of life, adapting to changing physical capacities and new psychological and social challenges. And they described mental health problems associated with failure to achieve milestones and objectives in their developmental schemes.

These theories have guided generations of psychodynamic therapists and child development experts. They are important to understand as the underpinnings of many therapeutic approaches, such as interpersonal therapy, some of which have been evaluated and found to be efficacious for some conditions. By and large, however, these theories have rarely been tested empirically.

Intellectual Development

The Swiss psychologist Jean Piaget also developed a

stage-constructed theory of children's intellectual development. Piaget's theory, based on several decades' observations of children (Inhelder & Piaget, 1958), was about how children gradually acquire the ability to understand the world around them through active engagement with it. He was the first to recognize that infants take an active role in getting to know their world and that children have a different understanding of the world than do adults. The principal limitations of Piaget's theories are that they are descriptive rather than explanatory. Furthermore, he neglected variability in development and temperament and did not consider the crucial interplay between a child's intellectual development and his or her social experiences (Bidell & Fischer, 1992).

Behavioral Development

Other approaches to understanding development are less focused on the stages of development. Behavioral psychology focused on observation and measurement, explaining development in terms of responses to stimuli, such as rewards. Not only did the theories of the early pioneers (e.g., Pavlov, Watson, and Skinner) generate a number of valuable treatments, but their focus on precise description set the stage for current programs of research based on direct observation. Social learning theory (Bandura, 1977) emphasized role models and their impact on children and adolescents as they develop. Several important clinical tools came out of behaviorism (e.g., reinforcement and behavior modification) and social learning theory (cognitive-behavioral therapy). Both treatment approaches are used effectively with children and adolescents.

Social and Language Development

Parent-Child Relationships

It is common knowledge that infants and, for the most part, their principal caretakers typically develop a close bond during the first year of life, and that in the second year of life children become distressed when they are forcibly separated from their mothers. However, the clinical importance of these bonds was not fully appreciated until John Bowlby introduced the concept of *attachment* in a report on the effects of maternal deprivation (Bowlby, 1951). Bowlby (1969) postulated that the pattern of an infant's early attachment to parents would form the basis for all later social relationships. On the basis of his experience with disturbed children, he hypothesized that, when the mother was unavailable or only partially available during the first months of the child's life, the attachment process would be interrupted, leaving enduring emotional scars and predisposing a child to behavioral problems.

A mother's bond with her child often starts when she feels fetal movements during pregnancy. Immediately after birth, most, but by no means all, mothers experience a surge of affection that is followed by a feeling that the baby belongs to them. This experience may not occur at all or be delayed under conditions of addiction or postnatal depression (Robson & Kumar, 1980; Kumar, 1997). Yet, like all enduring relationships, it seems that the relationship between mother and child develops gradually and strengthens over time. Some infants who experience severe neglect in early life may develop mentally and emotionally without lasting consequences, for example, if they are adopted and their adoptive parents provide sensitive, stable, and enriching care, or if depressed or substance-abusing mothers recover fully (Koluchova, 1972; Dennis, 1973; Downey & Coyne, 1990). Unfortunately, however, early neglect is all too often the precursor of later neglect. When the child remains subject to deprivation, inadequate or insensitive care, lack of affection, low levels of stimulation, and poor education over long periods of time, later adjustment is likely to be severely compromised (Dennis, 1973; Curtiss, 1977).

In general, it appears that the particular caregiver with whom infants interact (i.e., biological mother or another) is less important for the development of good social relationships than the fact that infants interact over a period of time with someone who is familiar and sensitive (Lamb, 1975; Bowlby, 1988). One of the problems in the later development of children who experience early institutionalization or significant neglect is that there may have been no opportunities for the caretakers and the infants to establish strong and mutual attachments in a reciprocating relationship.

Origins of Language

Recent research has established that successful use of language and communication is a cornerstone of childhood mental health. Not only are strong language capabilities critical to the development of such skills as listening and speaking, but they also are fundamental to the acquisition of proficient reading and writing abilities. In turn, children with a variety of speech and language impediments are at increasing risk as their language abilities fall behind those of their peers. Caretaker and baby start to communicate with each other vocally as well as visually during the first months of life. Many, but not all, developmental psychologists believe that this early pattern of mother-infant reciprocity and interchange is the basis on which subsequent language and communication develop. Various theorists have attempted to explain the relations between language and cognitive development (Vygotsky, 1962; Chomsky, 1965, 1975, 1986; Bruner, 1971; Luria, 1971), but no single theory has achieved preeminence. While a number of theories address language development from different perspectives, all theories suggest that language development depends on both biological and socio-environmental factors. It is clear that language competence is a critical aspect of children's mental health.

Relationships With Other Children

To be healthy, children must form relationships not only with their parents, but also with siblings and with peers. Peer relationships change over time. In the toddler period, children's social skills are very limited; they spend most of their time playing side by side rather than with each other in a give-and-take fashion.

As children grow, their abilities to form close relationships become highly dependent on their social skills. These include an ability to interpret and understand other children's nonverbal cues, such as body language and pitch of voice. Children whose social skills develop optimally respond to what other children say, use eye contact, often mention the other child's name, and may use touch to get attention. If they want to do something that other children oppose, they can articulate the reasons why their plan is a good one. They can suppress their own wishes and desires to reach a compromise with other children and may be willing to change—at least in the presence of another child—a stated belief or wish. When they are with a group of children they do not know, they are quiet but observant until they have a feeling for the structure and dynamics of the group (Coie & Kuperschmidt, 1983; Dodge, 1983; Putallaz, 1983; Dodge & Feldman, 1990; Kagan et al., 1998).

In contrast, children who lack such skills tend to be rejected by other children. Commonly, they are withdrawn, do not listen well, and offer few if any reasons for their wishes; they rarely praise others and find it difficult to join in cooperative activities (Dodge, 1983). They often exhibit features of oppositional defiant or conduct disorder, such as regular fighting, dominating and pushing others around, or being spiteful (Dodge et al., 1990). Social skills improve with opportunities to mix with others (Bridgeman, 1981). In recent years, knowledge of the importance of children's acquisition of social skills has led to the development and integration of social skills training components into a number of successful therapeutic interventions.

Temperament

During the past two decades, as psychologists began to view the child less as a passive recipient of environmental input but rather as an active player in the process, the importance of temperament has become better appreciated (Plomin, 1986). Temperament is defined as the repertoire of traits with which each child is born; this repertoire determines how people react to the world around them. Such variations in characteristics were first described systematically by Anna Freud from her observations of children orphaned by the ravages of World War II. She noticed that some children were affectionate, some wanted to be close but were too shy to approach adults, and some were difficult because they were easily angered and frustrated (A. Freud, 1965).

The first major longitudinal observations on temperament were begun in the 1950s by Thomas and Chess (1977). They distinguished 10 aspects of temperament, but there appear to be many different ways to describe temperamental differences (Goldsmith et al., 1987). Although there is some continuity in temperamental qualities throughout the life span (Chess & Thomas, 1984; Mitchell, 1993), temperament is often modified during development, particularly by the interaction with the caregiver. For example, a timid child can become bolder with the help of parental encouragement (Kagan, 1984, 1989). Some traits of temperament, such as attention span, goal orientation, lack of distractibility, and curiosity, can affect cognitive functioning because the more pronounced these traits are, the better a child will learn (Campos et al., 1983). Of note, it is not always clear whether extremes of temperament should be considered within the spectrum of mental disorder or whether certain forms of temperament might predispose a child to the development of certain disorders of brain .

Developmental Psychopathology

A number of central concepts and guiding assumptions underpin our current understanding of children's mental health and illness. These have been variously defined by different investigators (Sroufe & Rutter, 1984; Cicchetti & Cohen, 1995; Jensen, 1998), but by and large these tenets are based on the premise that psychopathology in childhood arises from the complex, multilayered interactions of specific characteristics of the child (including biological, psychological, and genetic factors), his or her environment (including parent, sibling, and family relations, peer and neighborhood factors, school and community factors, and the larger social-cultural context), and the specific manner in which these factors interact with and shape each other over the course of development. Thus, an understanding of a child's particular history and past experiences (including biologic events affecting brain development) is essential to unravel the why's and wherefore's of a child's particular behaviors, both normal and abnormal.

While this principle assumes developmental continuities, to the extent that early experiences are"brought forward" into the current behavior, it is also important to consider developmental discontinuities, where qualitative shifts in the child's biological, psychological, and social capacities may occur. These may not be easily discerned or predicted ahead of time and may reflect the emergence of new capacities (or incapacities) as the child's psychological self, brain, and social environment undergo significant reorganization.

A second precept underlying an adequate understanding of children's mental health and illness concerns the innate tendencies of the child to adapt to his or her environment. This principle of adaptation incorporates and acknowledges children's "self-righting" and"self-organizing" tendencies; namely, that a child within a given context naturally adapts (as much as possible) to a particular ecological niche, or when necessary, modifies that niche to get needs met. When environments themselves are highly disordered or pathological, children's adaptations to such settings may also be pathologic, especially when compared with children's behaviors within more healthy settings. This principle underscores the likelihood that some (but not all)"pathologic" behavioral syndromes might be best characterized as adaptive responses when the child or adolescent encounters difficult or adverse circumstances. Notably, this ability to adapt behaviorally is reflected at multiple levels, including the level of brain and nervous system structures (sometimes called neuroplasticity).

A third consideration that guides both research-based and clinical approaches to understanding child mental health and illness concerns the importance of age and timing factors. For example, a behavior that may be quite normal at one age (e.g., young children's distress when separated from their primary caretaking figure) can be an important symptom or indicator of mental illness at another age. Similarly, stressors or risk factors may have no, little, or profound impact, depending on the age at which they occur and whether they occur alone or with other accumulated risk factors.

A fourth premise underpinning an adequate understanding of children's mental health and illness concerns the importance of the child's context. Perhaps the most important context for developing children is their caretaking environment. Research with both humans and animals has demonstrated that gross disruptions in this critical parameter have immediate and long-term effects, not just on the young organism's later social-emotional development but also on physical health, long-term morbidity and mortality, later parenting practices, and even behavioral outcomes of its offspring. Moreover, context may play a role in the definition of what actually constitutes psychopathology or health. The same behavior in one setting or culture might be acceptable and even"normative," whereas it may be seen as pathological in another.

Yet another principle central to understanding child mental health and illness is that normal and abnormal developmental processes are often separated only by differences of degree. Thus, supposed differences between normal and abnormal behavior may be better understood by taking into account the differences in the amount or degree of the particular behavior, or the degree of exposure to a particular risk factor. Frequently, no sharp distinctions can be made.

The virtue of these developmental considerations when applied to children is that (a) they enable a broader, more informed search for factors related to the onset of, maintenance of, and recovery from abnormal forms of child behavior; (b) they help move beyond static diagnostic terms that tend to reduce the behaviors of a complex, developing, adapting, and feeling child to an oversimplified diagnostic term; (c) they offer a new perspective on potential targets for intervention, whether child-focused or directed toward environmental or contextual factors; and (d) they highlight the possibility of important timing considerations: windows of opportunity during a child's development when preventive or treatment interventions may be especially effective.

In the sections that follow, these considerations will help the reader understand the important differences from chapters focusing principally on adults, as well as the unique opportunities for intervention that occur because of these differences.

REVIEW QUESTIONS

1. What is normal development?
2. Which are the different theories of development
3. Who propounded the theory of Intellectual Development?

4. Elucidate social and language development among children.
5. What is behavioural development?
6. Explain the origins of languages.
7. What do you understand by "temperament"?
8. What is developmental psychopathology?

3

Adults and Mental Health

Mental health in adulthood is characterized by the successful performance of mental function, enabling individuals to cope with adversity and to flourish in their education, vocation, and personal relationships. These are the areas of functioning most widely recognized by the mental health field. Yet, from the perspective of different cultures, these measures may define the concept of mental health too narrowly. Many groups, particularly ethnic and racial minority group members, also emphasize community, spiritual, and religious ties as necessary for mental health. The mental health profession is becoming more aware of the importance of reaching out to other cultures; an innovation termed "linguistically and culturally competent services" is pertinent both to the field's conception of mental health and to the diagnosis and treatment of mental disorders.

An assortment of traits or personal characteristics have been viewed as contributing to mental health, including self-esteem, optimism, and resilience (Alloy & Abramson, 1988; Seligman, 1991; Institute of Medicine [IOM], 1994; Beardslee & Vaillant, 1997). These and related traits are seen as sources of personal resilience needed to weather the storms of stressful life events.

Stressful life events in adulthood include the breakup of intimate romantic relationships, death of a family member or friend, economic hardship, role conflict, work overload, racism and discrimination, poor physical health, accidental injuries, and intentional assaults on physical safety (Holmes

& Rahe, 1967; Lazarus & Folkman, 1984; Kreiger et al., 1993). Stressful life events in adulthood also may reflect past events. Severe trauma in childhood, including sexual and physical abuse, may persist as a stressor into adulthood, or may make the individual more vulnerable to ongoing stresses (Browne & Finkelhor, 1986). Although some kinds of stressful life events are encountered almost universally, certain demographic groups have greater exposure and/or vulnerability to their cumulative impact. These groups include women, younger adults, unmarried adults, African Americans, and individuals of lower socioeconomic status.

Anxiety disorders are the most prevalent mental disorders in adults (Regier et al., 1990). The anxiety disorders affect twice as many women as men. A broad category, anxiety disorders include panic disorder, phobias, obsessive-compulsive disorder, post-traumatic stress disorder, and generalized anxiety disorder, among others. Underlying this heterogeneous group of disorders is a state of heightened arousal or fear in relation to stressful events or feelings. The biological manifestations of anxiety, which are grounded in the "fight-or-flight" response, are unmistakable: they include surge in heart rate, sweating, and tensing of muscles. But this is certainly not the whole picture. Although the full array of biological causes and correlates of anxiety are not yet in our grasp, numerous effective treatments for anxiety disorders exist now. Treatment draws on an assortment of psychosocial and pharmacological approaches, administered alone or in combination.

Mood disorders take a monumental toll in human suffering, lost productivity, and suicide. Moreover, when unrecognized, they can result in unnecessary health care use. Mood disorders rank among the top 10 causes of *worldwide* disability (Murray & Lopez, 1996). Major depression and bipolar disorder are the most familiar mood disorders, but there are others including cyclothymia (alternating manic and depressive states that, while protracted, do not meet criteria for bipolar disorder) and dysthymia (a chronic, albeit symptomatically milder form of depression). The causes of mood disorders are not fully known. They may be triggered by stressful life events and enduring stressful social conditions (e.g., poverty and discrimination). With the exception of bipolar disorder, they too, like the anxiety disorders, are twice as common in women as men. One subtype of mood disorder, seasonal affective disorder, in which episodes of depression tend to occur in the late fall and winter, is seven times more common in women than in men (Blumenthal, 1988).

Mood disorders, like anxiety disorders, can be treated with a host of effective pharmacological and psychosocial treatments. Either type of treatment is effective for about 50 to 70 percent of patients in outpatient settings (Depression Guideline Panel, 1993). Severe depression seems to resolve more quickly with pharmacotherapy (Depression Guideline Panel, 1993) and may be helped further by multimodal therapy (the combination of pharmacotherapy and psychotherapy) (Thase et al., 1997b). Despite the efficacy of treatment, a surprising fraction of those with mood disorders go untreated (Katon et al., 1992; Narrow et al., 1993; Wells et al., 1994; Thase, 1996). The foremost barriers to treatment include cost, stigma, and problems in the organization of service systems that contribute to the underrecognition of these disorders.

Schizophrenia affects about 1 percent of the population, yet its severity and persistence reverberate throughout the mental health service system. Schizophrenia is marked by profound alterations in cognition and emotion. Symptoms frequently include hearing internal voices or experiencing other sensations not connected to an obvious source (hallucinations) and assigning unusual significance or meaning to normal events or holding false personal beliefs (delusions).

The course of illness in schizophrenia is quite variable, with most people having periods of exacerbation and remission. Schizophrenia had once been thought to have a uniformly downhill course, but recent research dispels this view. Long-term followup studies show that many individuals with schizophrenia significantly improve and some recover (Ciompi, 1980; Harding et al., 1992). Although the causes of schizophrenia are not fully known, research points to the prominent role of genetic factors and to the impact of adverse environmental influences during early brain development (Tsuang et al., 1991; Weinberger & Lipska, 1995; Andreasen, 1997b). New pharmacological treatments are at least as effective as past pharmacological treatments with fewer troubling side effects.

Effective treatment of schizophrenia extends well beyond pharmacological therapy: it also includes psychosocial interventions, family interventions, and vocational and psychosocial rehabilitation. For those patients who are high service users, treatment should be coordinated by an interdisciplinary team that provides high-intensity, community-based services (Lehman & Steinwachs, 1998a). The prototype for this intensive case-management approach, which is useful for persons with other severe and persistent mental disorders as well, is assertive community treatment, described more thoroughly later in this chapter. Among the services included in this approach is substance abuse treatment. Its inclusion stems from findings that about *half* of patients with serious mental disorders (including schizophrenia) develop alcohol or other drug abuse problems (Drake & Osher, 1997). Even though research generated a range of recommendations for effective treatment of schizophrenia, it is alarming that less than 50 percent of patients actually receive many of the recommended treatments and that the gap was more pronounced in African Americans (Lehman & Steinwachs, 1998b).

The social consequences of serious mental disorders—family disruption, loss of employment and housing—can be calamitous. Comprehensive treatment, which includes services that exist outside the formal treatment system, is crucial to ameliorate symptoms, assist recovery, and, to the extent that these efforts are successful, redress stigma. Consumer self-help programs, family self-help, advocacy, and services for housing and vocational assistance complement and supplement the formal treatment system. Many of these services are operated by consumers, that is, people who use mental health services themselves. The logic behind their leadership in delivery of these services is that consumers are thought to be capable of engaging others with mental disorders, serving as role models, and increasing the sensitivity of service systems to the needs of people with mental disorders (Mowbray et al., 1996).

Mental Health in Adulthood

What constitutes mental health during the adult years? A widely used standard of mental health is the *absence* of a defined mental disorder. This standard has its limitations (discussed later), yet remains useful for epidemiological purposes. Epidemiology studies investigate the prevalence of mental disorders within several time frames: current, the past 12 months, and across a lifetime. Two well-designed national epidemiologic surveys estimate that about 80 percent of the adult population of the United States do not have a mental disorder during a year and hence may be considered "mentally healthy" (i.e., absence of a mental disorder) during any given year (Regier et al., 1993; Kessler et al., 1994). Thus, the popular notion that *everyone* is "dysfunctional" is far from the truth. Yet, from time to time, many adults experience mental health problems.

Defining mental health by the absence of mental disorder does not convey the full picture of mental health. Among its limitations, this definition excludes adults with mental disorders who function well between episodes of illness. These people often are considered by themselves, and by coworkers, friends, and families, to be "mentally healthy" in spite of a history of mental illness and the risk of recurrence.

In addition to the mental health criteria cited earlier—that is, the successful performance of mental function, enabling individuals to cope with adversity and to flourish in their education, vocation, and personal relationships—a complementary approach defines the positive features of mental health in terms of attaining developmental milestones of adulthood, or in terms of displaying selected personality characteristics, traits, or attributes. Developmental theorist Erik Erikson viewed mental health in adulthood as achieving developmental tasks or milestones. According to Erikson's formulation and his subsequent empirical research on adult men, adulthood was the time for overcoming what he termed "psychosocial crises," the resolution of which led to satisfactory interpersonal and sexual relationships and to the pursuit of broader concerns for society and future generations (Erikson, 1963; Vaillant, 1977). However, these milestones, and the developmental theories that underpin them, have been criticized as reflecting the norms of European males rather than of women and other cultures.

Personality Traits

Mental health and mental illness can be seen as the product of various personality traits, behavior patterns, and other characteristics which have roots in the individual's prior life experiences or biology.

Personality traits are thought to confer either beneficial or detrimental effects on mental health during adulthood. Here too, however, there may be insufficient attention to gender and culture. The culture-bound nature of much of behavior has limited widespread predictive validity of personality research. (Mischel & Shoda, 1968). With this caveat in mind, a brief summary of healthy and maladaptive characteristics follows.

TABLE 1

Best estimate 1-year prevalence based on ECV and NCS, ages 18-54

	ECA Prevalence (%)	*NCS Prevalence (%)*	*Best Estimate ** (%)*
Any Anxiety Disorder	13.1	18.7	16.4
Simple Phobia	8.3	8.6	8.3
Social Phobia	2.0	7.4	2.0
Agoraphobia	4.9	3.7	4.9
GAD	(1.5)*	3.4	3.4
Panic Disorder	1.6	2.2	1.6
OCD	2.4	(0.9)*	2.4
PTSD	(1.9)*	3.6	3.6
Any Mood Disorder	7.1	11.1	7.1
MD Episode	6.5	10.1	6.5
Unipolar MD	5.3	8.9	5.3
Dysthymia	1.6	2.5	1.6
Biopolar I	1.1	1.3	1.1
Biopolar II	0.6	0.2	0.6
Schizophrenia	1.3	—	1.3
Nonaffective Psychosis	—	0.2	0.2
Somatization	0.2	—	0.2
ASP 2.1	—	2.1	
Anorexia Nervosa	0.1	—	0.1
Severe Cognitive Impairment	1.2	—	1.2
Any Disorder	19.5	23.4	21.0

*Numbers in parentheses indicate the prevalence of the disorder without any comorbidity. These rates were calculated using the NCS data for GAD and PTSD, and the ECA data for OCD. The rates were not used in calculating the any anxiety disorder and any disorder totals for the ECA and NCS columns. The unduplicated GAD and PTSD rates were added to the best estimate total for any anxiety disorder (3.3%) and any disorder (1.5%).

**In developing best-estimate 1-year prevalence rates from the two studies, a conservative procedure was followed that had previously been used in an independent scientific analysis comparing these two data sets (Andrews, 1995). For any mood disorder and any anxiety disorder, the lower estimate of the two surveys was selected, which for these data was the ECA. The best estimate rates for the individual mood and anxiety disorders were then chosen from the ECA only, in order to maintain the relationships between the individual disorders. For other disorders that were not covered in both surveys, the available estimate was used.

Key to abbreviations:

ECA, Epidemiologic Catchment Area;

NCS, National Comorbidity Study;

GAD, generalized anxiety disorder;

OCD, obsessive-compulsive disorder;

PTSD, post-traumatic stress disorder;

MD, major depression;

ASP, antisocial personality disorder.

Source: D. Regier, W. Narrow, & D. Rae, personal communication, 1999

Self-Esteem

Self-esteem refers to an abiding set of beliefs about one's own worth, competence, and abilities to relate to others (Vaughan & Oldham, 1997). Self-esteem also has been conceptualized as buffering the individual from adverse life events. Emotional well-being is often associated with a slightly positive, yet realistic, outlook (Alloy & Abramson, 1988). The opposite outlook is characterized by pessimism, demoralization, or minor symptoms of anxiety and depression. One seminal aspect of self-esteem has garnered much research attention: self-efficacy (Bandura, 1977). Self-efficacy is defined as confidence in one's own abilities to cope with adversity, either independently or by obtaining appropriate assistance from others. Self-efficacy is a major component of the construct known as resilience (i.e., the ability to withstand and overcome adversity). Other components of resilience include intelligence and problem solving, although resilience is also facilitated by having adequate social support (Beardslee & Vaillant, 1997).

Neuroticism

Neuroticism is a construct that refers to a broad pattern of psychological, emotional, and psychophysiologic reactivity (Eysenck & Eysenck, 1975). The opposite of neuroticism is stability or equanimity, which are major components of mental health. A high level of neuroticism is associated with a predisposition toward recognizing the dangerous, harmful, or defeating aspects of a situation and the tendency to respond with worry, anticipatory anxiety, emotionality, pessimism, and dissatisfaction. Neuroticism is associated with a greater risk of early-onset depressive and anxiety disorders (Clark et al., 1994). Neuroticism also may be linked to a particular cognitive attributional style in which life events are perceived to be large in impact and more difficult to change (Alloy et al., 1984). For example, this attributional style is embodied by pessimists who see every setback or failure as lasting forever, undermining everything, and being their fault (Seligman, 1991). Neuroticism also is associated with more rigid or distorted attitudes and beliefs about one's competence (Beck, 1976).

Avoidance

Avoidance describes an exaggerated predisposition to withdraw from novel situations and to avoid personal challenges as threats. This is the behavioral state that often accompanies the distress of someone who has a high level of neuroticism and low self-efficacy (Vaughan & Oldham, 1997). Closely related to the characteristics of behavioral inhibition or introversion, the trait of avoidance appears to be partly inherited and is associated with shyness, anxiety, and depressive disorders in both childhood and adult life, as well as the subsequent development of substance abuse disorders (Vaughan & Oldham, 1997; Kagan et al., 1988). The people with low levels of harm avoidance are described as "healthy extroverts" and are characterized by confident, carefree, or outgoing behaviors.

Impulsivity

Impulsivity is a trait that is associated with poor modulation of emotions, especially anger, difficulty delaying gratification, and novelty seeking. There is some developmental continuity between high levels of impulsivity in childhood and several adult mental disorders, including attention deficit hyperactivity disorder, bipolar disorder, and substance abuse disorders (Svrakic et al., 1993; Rothbart & Ahadi, 1994). Impulsivity also is associated with physical abuse (both as victim and, subsequently, as perpetrator) and antisocial personality traits (Vaughan & Oldham, 1997).

Sociopathy

This set of traits and behaviors refers to the predisposition to engage in dishonest, hurtful, unfaithful, and at times dangerous conduct to benefit one's own ends. The opposite of sociopathy may be referred to as character or scrupulosity. In its full form, sociopathy is referred to as antisocial personality disorder (DSM-IV). Sociopathy is characterized by a tendency and ability to disregard laws and rules, difficulties reciprocating within empathic and intimate relationships, less internalization of moral standards (i.e., a weaker conscience or superego), and an insensitivity to the needs and rights of others. People scoring high in sociopathy often have problems with aggressivity and are overrepresented among criminal populations. Although not invariably associated with criminality, sociopathy is associated with problematic, unethical, and morally questionable conduct in the workplace and within social systems. Marked sociopathy is much more common among men than women, although several other disorders (borderline and histrionic personality disorders and somatization disorder) are overrepresented among women within the same families (Widiger & Costa, 1994).

In summary, the various traits and behavioral patterns that epitomize strong mental health do not, of course, exist in a vacuum: they develop in a social context, and they underpin people's ability to handle psychological and social adversity and the exposure to stressful life events. Furthermore, severe or repeated trauma during youth may have enduring effects on both neurobiological and psychological development, altering stress responsivity and adult behavior patterns. Perhaps the best documented evidence of such enduring effects has been shown in young adults who experienced severe sexual or physical abuse in childhood. These individuals experience a greatly increased risk of mood, anxiety, and personality disorders throughout adult life.

REVIEW QUESTIONS

1. Explain the chief characteristics of mental health among adults.
2. What are anxiety disorders prevalent among adults?
3. What is mood disorders?
4. Write a note on mental health in adulthood.

4

Intelligence and Mental Processes

Intellectual development is, perhaps, one of the most misunderstood areas of child psychology. Although parents and teachers both use the term I.Q. (Intelligence Quotient) frequently they usually exhibit an unawareness of fundamental concepts regarding intelligence. Some people, for example, equate high intelligence and the capacity to do school work. They often ask the question, Why does Rohan who has a high I.Q. function poorly in school?" They assume that an intelligence test score is a complete predictor, encompassing motivational, emotional, and personality factors. A single score in a psychological study cannot tell us much about an individual; it is meaningful only in relationship to the total set of factors.

All teachers need help in learning to analyse the meaning of test scores more effectively. There has been far too much unsophisticated utilisation of both intelligence test and achievement test scores in the classroom. The scores can provide us with a measure of individual differences in performance in certain instances, but a single score should not be used to predict the potential of a given individual or to make permanent educational decisions. Perhaps a good policy for all teachers would be to recognise that test scores are most effectively utilised in the classroom in conjunction with other types of data. The teacher should also consider the child's personality, social development, physical makeup, concept of self as an achieving individual, and the way he has chosen to adjust to classroom expectations.

What do we mean when we talk about intelligence? Is there only one kind, or are there several kinds of intelligence? Is the IQ constant, or does it fluctuate? How much is the IQ influenced by heredity, how much by environment, and what can an individual do to improve the IQ scores of a given set of children? Are cultural factors present which prevent the child from scoring as well as he might? Does the "culture-free," "culture-fair" test really eliminate the factor of inequality of experience, and if we get a "culture-free" test, what kind of prediction does it give of functioning in schools that are closely tied to the culture? How is intelligence measured, and how often should it be measured in the schools? Is it possible for a child to raise his IQ through a change of environment, tutoring, intensive study, cramming, travel, and other types of experiences? How do emotions affect the intellect? Is it possible for emotional instability to affect the intelligence score?

The concept of intelligence has a variety of meanings, which are difficult to reduce to one simple definition. Intelligence has been defined as the ability to carry on abstract thinking, the ability to generalise, and the method of response to a problem situation.

Since Alfred Binet stimulated more psychological research studies on intelligence than any other single psychologist, perhaps we should begin with his definition of intelligence. Binet believed that intelligence was a combination of capacities that enabled the individual to adapt and be self-critical. In his general-factor theory, he included the abstract, mechanical, and social areas of behaviour as part of intelligence. Binet was concerned originally with establishing an accurate diagnosis of the intelligence of the retarded. His task was to determine whether certain students were ready for school experiences. In his tests, Binet stressed the examination of all types of capacities in order to determine criteria for stating that a child lacks the capacity to do scholastic work. In his original tests, in France, in 1905, Binet emphasised the primary factors of reasoning, comprehension and judgment. He proposed to set up a scale of tests to measure the development of the mental processes. Among the processes he included memory, images, recall, and attention. He established an age-scale approach to intelligence and eventually began to include children at all levels of intelligence. Binet made a most significant contribution to the study of intelligence. The construction of the intelligence scale and the emphasis on individual differences made a lasting contribution to the measurement of intellect. The Binet test is based on an age-scale performance formula. The normal child passes all items at age six when he is six. The normal eight year' old has a mental age of eight, the normal ten year old a mental age of ten.

Lewis Terman at Stanford University revised these scales in 1916, 1937, and 1960. The scale at the six-year level investigates vocabulary, differences in the meaning of words, ability to pick out missing elements in a picture, number concepts, opposite analogies, and maze tracing. Terman first translated, revised, and published in 1916 a Stanford revision of the Binet-Simon test to be used in English-speaking cultures. In this work Terman defined intelligence as the ability to carry on abstract thinking and to utilise abstract symbols in the solution of problems. Terman's research seemed to indicate that vocabulary was the best single indicator of an individual's general intelligence. Terman's revision of the Binet was redone in 1937 and then again, posthumously, in 1960; it provided psychology with an extremely useful predictor of the capacity to utilise abstract symbols in a variety of cultural settings.

It must be remembered here that not all psychologists have accepted Binet's and Terman's definitions of intelligence. Some have developed intelligence scales based on different assumptions, such as the Wechsler and Thurstone assumptions.

Charles E. Spearman began the transition from the general-factor theory to multiple-factor analysis, through his development of a two-factor theory of human capacity. He called the two factors involved in the intellectual performance of a task "G" and "S." "G" underlies all mental functioning and is considered the common denominator in all sorts of mental performance. This factor varies from individual to individual but is consistent in all aspects of a given individual's mental functioning. Since mental functioning in unrelated situations calls for different types of mental accomplishments, a specific factor must also operate in each situation. The factor "S" varies not only from individual to individual, but also within the individual, i.e., intraindividual variability.

L.L. Thurstone was an important figure in the early development of factor analysis. He believed that a single intelligence index was inadequate for the purpose of describing mental capacities. He believed that a great many factors entered into specific skills in a variety of combinations. Multiple-factor analysis was designed to discover and isolate fundamental human traits, and Thurstone was able to isolate the following factors: ability to verbalise, word fluency, number facility, memory, visualising or space thinking, perceptual speed, induction, and speed of judgment. The results of Thurstone's Analysis of Intelligence appears in the Primary Abilities Test (PMA) published by Science Research Associates.

The 1963 edition of the PMA covers grades K-1, 2-4, 4-6, 6-9, and 912. The purpose of the test is to investigate primary mental abilities considered most significant in schoolwork. As defined in the manual, the five primary abilities measured by the test are:

V—Verbal Meaning

The ability to understand ideas expressed in words. In the later school years this is the most important single index of a child's potential for handling academic tasks. At the lower levels it is tested by a vocabulary test in picture form; at the upper levels, by a verbal vocabulary test.

N—Number Facilit:

The ability to work with numbers, to handle simple quantitative problems rapidly and accurately, and to understand and recognise quantitative differences. At the lower-grade levels, the N scores are determined by a pictorial test that requires no reading. Addition problems are also used. At the upper levels, arithmetical reasoning problems are included.

R—Reasoning

The ability to solve logical problems. Separate measures of this ability are not provided in the batteries designed for grades K through 4. In the 4-6 battery it is measured by word-grouping and figure-grouping tests; at the upper levels, by word-grouping, letter-series, and number-series tests.

P—Perceptual Speed

The ability to recognise likenesses and differences between objects or symbols quickly and accurately. This ability is important in acquiring reading skills but tends to plateau at a relatively early age. For this reason it is included only with the three batteries designed for the lower grades.

S—Spatial Relations

The ability to visualise objects and figures rotated in space and the relations between them. The test measuring this ability appears in every level of the PMA and is important throughout the school years.

Numerous psychologists have suggested that there are really different kinds of intelligence. Thorndike said intelligence might be divided into three areas-abstract intelligence, or the ability to deal with the symbolic, e.g., a word, a code, or a geometric figure; mechanical intelligence, or the ability to deal with concrete objects; and social intelligence, the use of psychological principles involving problems of human relationships.

J.P. Guilford has attempted through factor analysis to develop a unified theory of intelligence. He defines a factor as a unique ability needed to do well in a particular class of tasks. Guilford devised a theoretical model of one hundred twenty cells. each of which represents a distinct ability. In his model, the factors are classified in three fundamental ways: processes, such as memory, cognition, divergent production, convergent production; contents or materials, such as symbolic, semantic and behavioural; and products, result of applying a particular operation to content, including units, relations, and systems.

Guilford speaks of several kinds of intelligence. Concrete intelligence enables one to use figural information: abstract intelligence affects abilities pertaining to both symbolic and semantic content; and, finally, social intelligence, which enables one to work effectively with people. Thus, Guilford presents us with a background which might eventually be used in understanding the development and the measurement of intelligence.

From the phenomenological point of view, intelligence is a function of interaction. Intelligence is seen as dependent upon the richness and variety of perceptions possible for the individual at a given moment. Psychologists like Combs have pointed out that in most individuals the quality of perception hinges on the experiences the individual has accumulated. Combs believes that the quality of an individual's intelligence is affected by exposure to a wide variety of experiences that permit him to improve perception. Implicit in the perceptual approach is the belief that a person will not behave any more intelligently than he believes he can. A child who is convinced that he cannot do arithmetic and spelling or understand geography will act in accordance with his convictions. To enable him to utilise his capacities, his convictions must be changed. Intelligence then is considered as a product of the interaction of a person and his perceived psychological environment, and the intelligence test does not accurately measure the potential differentiations the individual can make, but his functional perceptions. The phenomenologist would, therefore, caution users to recognise the factors that limit perception, such as physical conditions, opportunity, experiences, exposure to symbolic events, and the individual's own goals and values.

MENTAL GROWTH

As a child develops, he makes increasingly complex adaptive responses to his physical and social environment. Mental development can be inferred from this behaviour. While children differ widely in both rate and pattern of mental development, developmental progression can be observed and, to an extent, measured.

Mental growth curves have been developed for infants. In one of the earlier studies of mental development, a group of thirty-one male and thirty female infants were studied. During the first two years of life yearly increases in point scores were noted, as shown in the accompanying graph. Scores indicate that the infants' mental development was rapid to about the ninth or tenth month, after which deceleration was evident.

Since tasks required on an infant test are of a motor and perceptual nature, behaviour growth in the early months of infant development has been demonstrated to have little predictive validity for the later tests of development of intelligence.

To understand individual mental development, it is necessary to study longitudinally the development of intelligence in individuals.

Curves derived from averages of the mental development of a group of children differ from repeated tests of individual children over a period of time.

In any study of mental development, we should always be cautious about inferring the rate of development from mental test scores. These scores do not represent absolute measurements, the size of which are necessarily equivalent at each point on the scale. For example, the year's mental development, even in the case of an average child, may not be the same between any two successive years. The intellectual increment between the ages four and five is not necessarily the same size as the increments between eight and nine or twelve and thirteen. We do not have an absolute scale for measurement in the intellectual area.

Intelligence in young children is measured by functions considerably different from those used to measure older children. Thus, it is obvious that the scales are far from equivalent. On the Binet a four year old is asked to identify objects in a picture vocabulary, name objects from memory, discriminate between forms, draw opposite analogies, and do simple comprehension items. At age eleven he would be required to produce a design from memory', comprehend verbal absurdities, define abstract words, memorise a sentence, solve problems, and indicate how certain objects are similar. The abilities being measured at eleven are somewhat different and cannot be assumed to be merely an extension or expansion of four year-old abilities.

Curves representing scores made on repeated administrations of tests may not reflect actual intellectual development. Courtis maintains that no single type of growth curve can adequately express the pattern of mental growth because of the nature of the items included on the typical intelligence test. These curves lack stability, he believes, because they do not measure a uniform function in a uniform manner. Courtis thinks adequate study of mental growth will come only when developmental progress in the performance of a single act is considered. Courtis indicates that we must get back to single-variable research if we are to study development accurately. Growth curves have value because they make it possible for us to note the child's rate of progress, spurts, plateaus, and regressions in relation to his unique pattern.

Researchers in mental development have attempted to determine the point of mental maturity when mental growth ceases. The finding of Terman and Merrill that mental age does not increase after the age of fifteen years has since been attributed to the limited ceiling on the 1937 Revision of the Stanford-Binet. Evidence based on a wider sample and retesting of the same population shows that the age of terminal growth may be twenty-five or even beyond. There are reports of gains in intelligence test scores at age twenty-five on the Wechsler-Bellvue, and even at age fifty on the Army Alpha and Concept Maturity Test.

Bayley studied five boys from the age of one month to twenty-five years. She found that each child had an individual pattern, and after the infancy period there was an underlying pattern of development constancy. These five boys were tested at twenty-five years of age and all had continued to improve in their Wechsler-Bellevue scores. Bayley indicates that the intellectual processes measured had not reached a ceiling, with fourteen out of fifteen participants continuing to show gains. Thus the issue of terminal growth in development of a cognitive process varies considerably from individual to individual.

Research in mental development has pointed to some general trends. During infancy and the preschool period, the abilities measured by intellignce tests are genrally perceptual and sensory-motor in nature. Following this early stage of development, the lementary school years use tests in which abstract intelligence tends to be most important. Abstract abilities are highly correlated. During predolescence and later on, tests show a considerable differentiation of intellectual abilities. Thurstone domonstrated a differential growth rate for mental abilities. Perception, reasoning, and space abilities develop somewhat earlier than numerical and momery abilities, while verbal abilities develop more slowly.

In its time, The Harvard Growth Study was probably one of the most comprehensive longitudinal studies in the field of physical and mental growth. Some of the conclusions of Dearborn and Rothney are significant for our study of intellectual growth

1. Physical and mental growth are essentially individual affairs. No two cases have been found to have exactly the same developmental history as indicated in terms of their deviation from the averages of groups of which they are members.
2. The relationship between physical measurements and mental measurements is so low that the knowledge of one does not enable us to predict the other.
3. The use of different mental tests over the years indicates that each test is characterised by its own single and peculiar differences with respect to the problems of practise effect and its relation to individual test problems.
4. The group mental tests used in this study yielded higher IQ's than the Stanford-Binet tests.

8. In general, children tend to remain throughout the period of their mental growth (to age sixteen) in the same classification as they were at age eight.
9. In general, individuals tend to Perform at the same level on verbal and non-verbal material which appears in group mental tests.
10. Complete substitution of non-verbal for verbal material in mental tests, would result in handicapping as many children as does the use of tests using verbal material only.

11. Mental growth, as measured by the type of group mental tests used in this study, continues much beyond the age of adolescence, although with markedly decreased rate after the age of twenty.
12. The possibility of using the percentage of growth based on the estimated maximum growth of the individual, or of an unselected group, in preference to the mental age technique, and the inadequacy of the commonly employed intelligence quotient, as an index of mental growth has been demonstrated.
13. The advantage of using individual growth curve constructed with the above described "growth unit" has been noted.
15. Performance on mental tests does not seem to be related in any way with pubescent growth spurt.

In a more recent analysis of the Harvard Growth Study, Ethel Cornell and Charles Armstrong found general patterns of mental growth occurred in spurts.

1. A single growth curve theoretically reaching maturity between the ages twenty-six and twenty-seven, maturity being indicated by a mean level of ability regarded as just above average.

2. Two growth curves—the earlier one terminating around age thirteen, the second one not becoming evident until age fifteen or sixteen, with maturity theoretically indicated at about twenty-three to twenty-four years of age, at a level slightly above average. (Female)

3. Two growth curves-most rapid development from nine to thirteen, the later period one of slow increase with maturity theoretically reached at age twenty-eight to twenty-nine years, at the highest mean level of ability of all the patterns. (Male)

Individual differences in mental growth are observed in early infancy. When compared to a group, the mental growth of children seems to remain at a fairly fixed position, unless some serious changes in conditions of development occur. The child who fails to grow consistently cannot be predicted. The growth curve of intelligence can be generalised, but without certainty because of individual differences in both rate and maximum.

Nancy Bayley pointed out some striking examples of variation in mental growth. One child in her study, Mark, varied from his highest score when tested at one month, to group norm at one year, to the lowest one-fourth at two years; he remained at this position relative to the group until age seven, then rose steadily until he received the following IQ scores: at nine years 117; at ten years 122; at twelve years 130. Gerald, the brightest six month old, was consistently slow from then on, scoring 85 at nine, 84 at ten and 76 at eleven. Charles rose from the twenty-fifth percentile at age one year to average intelligence at four years and scored 146, 149, and 153 at nine, ten, and eleven years of age. These scores would place him in the ninety-ninth percentile of the Stanford-Binet scale.

In the Berkeley Guidance Study, one girl rose from the thirty-first percentile at twenty-one months to the ninety-ninth at six years. Another at the same age dropped from the fifty-fourth to the sixth percentile. These extreme variations are not the rule, but they do show the danger of trying to predict the IQ, particularly in the early years.

The age at which an individual ceases to grow in intellectual ability may range from adolescence to the twenties. Increases in ability after the age of twenty appear to be horizontal-in other words, an extension of knowledge.

Our study of mental growth curves indicates the necessity

for a revised conception of intelligence by the schools and teachers. It seems reasonable to suggest that the research presented should shake the belief of those who tend to think that a single intelligence test will predict a mental growth pattern.

To speak of the constancy of the IQ without considering the many factors which affect this score at different age levels is to disadvantage a great percentage of the children. The use, in the elementary school, of IQ scores for the development of homogeneous groups becomes a particularly naive concept. Constancy of the IQ can now be disputed, and teachers, administrators, and psychologists would do well to consider problems involved both in the measurement of intelligence and the mental growth curves before attempting any early classification of individuals.

FACTORS INFLUENCING INTELLIGENCE

Physical and Hereditary Factors

A natural endowment unfolds maturationally and sets limits on potential intellectual functions. This native intellectual endowment varies among individuals, and its maturation is hindered or assisted by the type of stimulation available in the environment during the early years. By comparing increments in mental and physical growth in curves of mental and physical development, Abernethy found that rates of physical and mental growth were essentially unrelated within the normal range of individual differences. He believed that the entire period of development is involved in determining the small positive correlations typically found between physical and mental growth during childhood.

Olson and Hughes found a general correlation of all aspects of child growth when plotted according to derived age values.

Shuttleworth, who worked with data from the Harvard Growth Study, also found that both boys and girls with early maximum-growth ages in standing height proved to be more intelligent than children with late maximum-growth ages. His findings support the evidence of Abernethy, Olson, and Hughes that growth proceeds in patterned fashion.

Environmental and Cultural Factors

Investigations (conducted since the beginning of psychological research) tend to show that the higher the socioeconomic status, the higher the average intelligence of the children. The basic question is whether higher socioeconomic position helps to raise the level of intelligence or, more simply, whether intelligent people rise in the social scale? It has been demonstrated that the intellectual level of the underprivileged can be improved by raising their socioeconomic levels, especially if an early enough start is made. However, not every child gains and the degree of improvement varies greatly. The culturally rich home environment tends to lift the IQ, some believe as much as twenty points, while the home environment devoid of positive cultural influences, may lower the IQ as much as twenty points. More adequate research on this issue is still needed. Some problems obviously exist in failure of the tests to equate for cultural differences.

What does the upper socioeconomic group provide that results in a higher intelligence quotient? The most important factors appear to be nutrition, adequate medical attention, security (derived from freedom from economic deprivation), and exceptional educational advantages. A child, devoid of advantages in the area of food, clothing, physical and mental care, is frequently a culturally deprived child who scores low on the intelligence test. The most extensive documentation of the significance of experience in determining the growth of learning ability has been made by Hunt.

During World War II, armed services tested the intelligence of people from all sections of the country. Scores were found to parallel the amount of money per pupil spent on public schools in the various states. Men from states with high educational expenditures had the highest average IQ scores.

Some argue that tests favour the upper socioeconomic group. This argument is made particularly by people interested in developing the culture-fair tests.

The upper socioeconomic classes provide advantages, but psychologists believe that a "good psychological home" is more important than a home with just economic advantages, since every child has a unique set of nature and nurture experiences. The family atmosphere and family constellation for him are different from his brothers' and sisters'. The child has a distinct primary reactivity pattern and a capacity to use the nature and nurture factors in a distinct and unique manner.

The nature and nurture, or, hereditary and environment problem is not easily solved. Most research studies on this problem are inconclusive. The best conclusion to date is that the influences of heredity and environment are inextricably interwoven, and, hence, it cannot be demonstrated that one is a more significant factor than the other.

Emotional Factors

Richards studied the development of a disturbed boy, with an emphasis upon the relationship of intelligence-test performance at various ages to the child's life situation during the same period. He produced two sets of data, test scores and a history of the individual's adjustment at the time of each testing. The intelligence testing showed the following results on the Stanford-Binet at various ages: the average IQ for all testing was 124, the individual IQ's fluctuating between 117 and 140. There are four trends in the curve he obtained for IQ's between the ages of three and ten. First, a rise of eleven IQ points from age three to four, then a drop of thirteen points from five to six, a rise again of twenty-five points from six to eight years, and finally a drop of eighteen points from eight to ten years. The boy, referred to as Bobbie Jones, was studied at the Fels Research Institute. The Fels Parent Behaviour Scales were used several times throughout the years. Projectives tests such as the Rorchach and the Thematic Apperception Test were available.

Family Resemblances

A number of investigations on intelligence have explored the relationship between parents and their own children, parents and adopted children, twins, and siblings. Leahy noted that the coefficients correlation between intelligence in parents and adopted children correlated about .20 while coefficients for own children were generally found to be about .50. This might be considered a significant difference since adopted children are generally assigned by agencies on the basis of a fairly high relationship between the parents, the child, and the educational setting of the home.

Many studies have shown that in general we can demonstrate a correlation of about .50 between the intelligence of fathers or mothers and their children. This same approximate correlation has been found between siblings, who live in somewhat the same environment.

Correlations between the intelligence of identical twins who have developed from the same fertilised ovum usually range between .70 and .90. Newman, Freeman, and Holzinger found that the IQ's of twins who experienced the same environmental opportunities and education were on the whole closer than the IQ's of twins whose environment and education differed considerably. They also noted that identical twins who were reared apart were, as a group, more alike than siblings who were reared in the same home.

Honzik suggested that there is a significant relationship which changes with age between parental ability and the child's intelligence test scores. For example, she found a shift from a coefficient correlation of about .05 between mother and child at age two to a coefficient as high as .35 at age five and thereafter. Data from Skodak in the same figure show similar relationships between the adopted child's IQ and the true mother's education. Honzik concluded that the parent-child correlations reflect individual differences which are largely determined genetically.

Shields did a study of forty-four monozygotic, or one-egg twins with exactly the same hereditary equipment. He found a correlation on intelligence of .76 when these twins were reared together, a correlation of .77 when reared apart, and a correlation of .51 in dizygotic twins where hereditary equipment is not identical. This points to the strong influence of heredity.

School Factors

A basic question is the extent to which the child's intelligence is influenced by the type of schooling he receives and the time he receives it. There have been some investigations in connection with nursery school and the raising of a child's IQ. Olson and Hughes found that nursery school children from privileged backgrounds did not differ significantly in intellectual growth from nonnursery school children who also came from privileged backgrounds. Remember that these children came from homes where nursery school experiences could add little to the nurture of the child's intellectual development. In this study, then, no special intellectual effects were attributed to nursery school and kindergarten attendance for children who experienced adequate nurture in their own homes.

Tests are used not only to determine the present status of the individual but also to make predictions about his future growth and status. In order to make an effective educational decision, we need to have the best possible measures of intelligence available.

Anderson concluded that the prediction of later status from early test scores will be less accurate the younger the child is at the time of first testing or the longer the interval between tests.

After the appearance of speech in the child, tests begin to have greater predictive value. In general, it could be concluded that indices for prediction of future development are quite ineffective until the age of six or seven. Some of this ineffectiveness is due to the fact that infant intelligence tests deal with functions that are quite different from those on tests used during the elementary school years and adolescence. There are many reservations about items on the Gesell Schedule for predicting intellectual status which are administered prior to age two or even age five.

Intelligence is a developing function and the stability of measured intelligence increases with age. Bayley did a comprehensive study of the intellectual growth of forty children between ages one month and eighteen years of age, which showed wide differences in the growth patterns of individual children in the area of mental ability. The shifts were almost unpredictable, occurring at all age levels and in a wide range of abilities. In an article in the *American Psychologist*, in 1955, Bayley presented some of the different patterns of intellectual growth between one month and twenty-five years of age.

Growth of Intelligence

Factors have been identified as beneficial to the growth and development of intelligence. The psychological climate that the child is raised in is one of the most significant. The child needs to feel accepted and valued as an individual. His ideas; thoughts, and even idiosyncracies should be listened to, accepted, and discussed in a mature fashion. He should not be laughed at as immature because he has an idea that is different. Instead, a climate should be created in which having unique ideas and making contributions to family living are rewarded.

The implication is that the child must be encouraged to make choices, solve problems, and become independent in his thinking. This type of behaviour should always be reinforced and encouraged. It is also vital that the child be provided with materials and information which permit problem solving. He should be allowed to develop new uses for old tools, to see new relationships, to do creative writing, and to have access to a wide variety of experiences and hooks. The family needs to provide a system for the regular recognition of achievement in the intellectual area. There should be an atmosphere which provides stimulation for all kinds of broad intellectual growth and which permits the child to work on his developmental problems and developmental tasks. He should be made aware of the alternatives and then encouraged to solve the problem. Adults need to have faith that children can learn from the consequences of their decisions.

The growth of intelligence is dependent upon a stimulating atmosphere and a creative relationship with the significant adults both in the home and in the school.

Intelligence Measurement

Schools and placement agencies have been interested in the subject of intelligence testing because of its implications for placement. Intelligence tests attempt to predict the individual's capacity to function generally in tasks that require scholastic aptitude. They measure the individual's ability to cope with situations requiring the exercise of mental processes and try to measure the ability to comprehend the situation, apply past experiences, and solve the problem presented.

Tests are designed on the premise that intelligence can not be measured directly but is inferred by the observation or evaluation of behaviour. Behaviour has been grouped at various chronological age levels, and decisions have been made as to what is intelligent behaviour for a given age level. The measurements are converted into norms for representative groups of a population, so that eventually individuals can be classified as having intelligence like a typical five year old or eight year old. Some tests, like the Kuhlmann-Anderson, used a median score in an attempt to avoid the averaging of scores in determining the norms.

Most tests of intelligence place a premium on the ability to do abstract thinking through the use of symbols. Vocabulary also is of great importance in measuring intelligence. Many psychologists believe that as a child matures his vocabulary is the best single indicator of intelligence as related to scholastic aptitude. This measurement of vocabulary can be made in an individual test, such as the Stanford-Binet or the Wechsler Intelligence Scale for Children, or in group testing.

For a long time, test makers have been concerned with the problem of avoiding measuring only differences in cultural opportunities or education. An effective test item combines a criterion of novelty and universality. It is novel in the sense that it has not been encountered before by individuals taking the test; it is universal to the extent that all, at a certain level, may have had some experience related to it.

The group intelligence test has frequently been shown to have a high relationship to the extent, level, and quality of the child's educational experience. When we speak of measuring intellectual potential or "native capacity," therefore, we need to be aware of the overlapping of hereditary and environmental factors.

The teacher and school administrator must be aware of

some of the problems involved in the measurement of intelligence. We must not assume that tests with similar titles measure similar behaviours. We must always determine whether the group on which the norms for this test were based is comparable to the children we are testing. It is also pertinent to recognise that tests with dissimilar titles may actually measure the same thing. It is quite applicable in testing to ask, "What's in a name"" Intelligence testing with children must hold to a definite concept about what the test items are seeking to predict.

Psychologists engaged in test construction also need to recognise the cyclic nature of mental development. At certain times mental development proceeds more rapidly than at other times. Those who use intelligence tests in the schools should recognise that children with identical IQ's seldom function identically. One reason for this could very well be that they had acquired their mental-age points on different kinds of abilities and tasks.

Inhelder and Piaget also found differences in the modal age of children at a given stage on two different tasks. The age level for attainment of a given stage appears to be specific to a task rather than general, so that the child can operate at stage two on one task and at stage one on another.

The first individual intelligence test was the Stanford-Binet. Originally devised for use in dealing with a specific problem in France, it was later revised by Terman and then Terman and Merrill, and has been used extensively in the United States. The test items in this scale have been arranged in the order of empirically determined difficulty from the age of two upward. Items are always scored on a pass or fail basis. There are six test items at each half-year level from age two to five and six items at each yearly age level thereafter until the age of fourteen. Thereafter, the test provides for average and superior adult levels. The items have been arranged so that the normal child of a given age is expected to perform at his chronological-age level. Retarded children perform below the level, gifted children above.

Another frequently used individual intelligence test is the Wechsler Intelligence Scale for children (WISC), which the psychologist uses diagnostically to determine areas of strength and weakness. The Wechsler test, developed and originally copyrighted by David Wechsler in 1949, abandoned the concept of mental age originally introduced by Binet in 1908. The Wechsler test has instead worked on the basis of a deviation intelligence quotient. The IQ is obtained by comparing the child's test performance with the scores earned by individuals in a single age group, not with the composite age group. This was done in an attempt to keep the standard deviation of IQ's identical from year to year, so that a child's obtained IQ does not vary unless his actual test performance as compared with his peers varies. The Wechsler test also permits development of a verbal, performance, and total or full-scale intelligence quotient. The verbal factors include information, comprehension, arithmetic, similarities, vocabulary, and digit span. The performance factors include picture completion, picture arrangement, block design, object assembly, coding, and mazes.

Group intelligence tests are frequently used in the schools to make educational decisions. Close analysis reveals that many mental-ability tests being widely used are really strictly measures of classroom achievement, while others are quite independent of classroom instruction. The person who selects or uses tests needs to know whit the test actually measures. Individual deviations due to motivation, fatigue, distraction and the like may not be noted in a group-testing situation.

The following list includes some of the tests now being used in the public schools:

1. The California Test of Mental Maturity. Authors, E. T. Sullivan, W. W. Clark, end E. W. Tiegs. Publisher, California Test Bureau. Grades four to twelve.
2. Cattell Culture-fair Intelligence Test. Author, R. B. Cattell. Publisher, Bobbs-Merrill Co., Inc. School-learned skills not required. Grades three to twelve.
3. Differential Aptitude Tests. Authors, C. Bennett, H. Seashore, and A. Wesman. Publisher, Psychological Corporation. Items generally well-constructed and frequently used in grades eight to twelve to make educational and vocational decisions.
4. Lorge-Thorndike Intelligence Test. Authors, I. Lorge, R. L. Thorndike. Publisher, Houghton Mifflin Company. A promising instrument for predicting achievement in grade one. Series considered to be a well-constructed set of growth scales.
5. Science Research Associates Tests of General Ability (TOGA). Author, J. C. Flanagan. Publisher, Science Research Associates. Measures cultural understandings and reasoning with geometric forms.
6. Henmon-Nelson Tests of Mental Ability. Authors, T. A. Lanken, M. J. Nelson. Publisher, Houghton Mifflin Company. Places a. great emphasis on reading; scores tend to correlate well with teacher grades. Grades three to twelve.
7. Otis Quick Scoring Mental Ability Tests. Author, A. S. Otis. Publisher, Harcourt, Brace & World, Inc. Grades four to twelve. Places a great emphasis on school skills.
8. School and College Ability Tests (SCAT). Author, Educational Testing Service Staff. Publisher, Educational Testing Service. Grades four to twelve. A new test, which provides both a verbal and a quantitative score. Considered to be a good measure of school-learned abilities.

9. Kuhlman-Anderson Intelligence Tests. Authors, F. Kuhlman and R. G. Anderson. Publisher, Personnel Press. Grades three to twelve. Well-constructed and considered to be one of the better measures of growth available. Emphasises both reading and achievement skills.
10. S.R.A. Primary Ability Test. Grades four to twelve. Authors, L. L. Thurstone and T. C. Thurstone. Publisher, Science Research Associates. Grades four to twelve. Stresses reading, arithmetic arid reasoning abilities.

Because the testing held is frequently under attack from critics of education, it is important that the teacher and the parent understand more adequately the school testing programme and some of the significant concepts related to it. Robert Bauernfeind's *Building a School Testing Programme* (Boston: Houghton Mifflin Company, 1963) is recommended to those interested in investigating testing problems further.

Use of Test Results: An Interpretation

Individual tests permit a more reliable measure of intelligence than a group test. The motivation and effort produced are more uniform when the child works under the supervision of an examiner in a one-to-one relationship, and the examiner can observe the individual to determine if there is sustained effort and attention.

You should always be aware of the standard error of measurement for any test you use. For example, an IQ of 90 should never be thought of as exactly 90, but rather between 80 and 100. The instruments used for measurement are not precise, and the scores should not be taken as exact measurements.

Test results should be considered in terms of the reliability of the instrument. Has it been demonstrated that the test yields approximately the same result when applied to a number of children of the type you are concerned about? Also, is the test valid in the sense that it has accurately predicted the kind of precise information that you need for the decision you have to make? Are the norms representative of the characteristics of the group that the child being tested has to compete with? Are the size of the norm population and the recency of the sampling adequate?

A reading disability frequently affects IQ test performance on paper and pencil tests. Some evidence indicates that where reading is accelerated, the IQ is equally accelerated, whereas the child who is slow or retarded in reading may produce an intelligence score lower than his potential. Such factors as those related to reading can be checked out through the use of the individual test. It is also possible to give nonverbal tests to clarify the effects of a reading disability. The culture of the individual, his background, and previous set of experiences should always be considered to see whether they are comparable both to the norm group and to the groups with which he is currently competing.

In interpreting the results of tests, the culture and environmental opportunity of the child must be taken into consideration. The same score means one thing in a child from deprived circumstances and another in a child from a rich cultural environment. The teacher should remember that IQ's on group tests may measure abstract intelligence or scholastic aptitude and that this is only one type of ability. Group tests rarely measure the ability to work with things or with people, nor do they measure the ability to solve many concrete, practical problems. The child who scores low on group intelligence tests generally has trouble with academic work. However, he may have a good ability in mechanical, social, artistic, or other areas. Thus, tests may tell us not only what behaviour is present and what is not present but may give us clues for other types of investigation.

READINESS TESTING

A significant evaluation problem for the school is the widely varying capacities evident in the functioning of children as they enter kindergarten and first grade. An effective readiness test should provide the kind of information that makes it possible to adapt the educational programme to the individual. It is quite evident that capacities develop at different rates in different children and that chronological age is an extremely poor measure to attempt to correlate with any given ability. Although we accept the fact that children do not begin to speak or walk or sit up at the same age, our schools seem to assume that children are ready to learn on the basis of chronological-age factors.

Individual tests of readiness have received increasing attention. The Brenner-Gestalt Test is an example of an individual measure of school readiness. The test is comparatively brief, taking about 10 minutes to administer individually to each child, and measures whether the child is able to work with certain concrete number concepts. Does he recognise the number set of dots represents; can he count the number of dots in a given set? He is also asked to reproduce a sentence and to reproduce a Gestalt figure. The final part of the Brenner-Gestalt Test requires him to draw a man, Dr. Anton Brenner of the Merrill-Palmer Institute, Detroit, Michigan, has set up a scoring system and a set of standards to evaluate readiness for school work based on these measures.

Another individual measure of school readiness is the battery of tests developed by Frances Ilg and Louise Bates Ames of the Gesell Institute of Child Development. This test determines a developmental age by giving the child a battery of behaviour tests, including an interview; writing of name, address, letters, numbers; copy forms; Gesell incomplete-man test; right and left test; Munroe visual one and visual three; naming animals; giving home and school preferences;

Lowenfeld mosaic tests. Tables of norms for each test are also available. These tests are designed to be used at the entrance to both kindergarten and first grade. They are set up so as to project a total view of the child and his readiness for the varied tasks of school.

The revised Stanford-Binet has also been used frequently to determine readiness for school tasks. The Psychological Corporation has been interested in this problem and as a result has undertaken development of a test to measure intellectual functioning in children age four through six and one-half years, the period just :prior to formal schooling. In general, this new test is a downward revision of the WISC that operates as a distinct and separate scale. The Wechsler Preschool and Primary Scale of Intelligence consists of the following items: information, animal house, vocabulary, picture completion, arithmetic, mazes, sentences, geometric designs block designs, similarities, and comprehension.

THE GIFTED CHILD

For our purposes we shall consider the child who has consistently scored an IQ of 130 or more as gifted. We would also like to expand the concept to include any child who shows exceptional performance in any worthwhile function. Thus, giftedness might include not only the intellectually talented, but those with promise in mechanics, music, linguistics, social capacities, and artistic and physical areas, as well as the intellectually talented. Certainly it would include dramatics and creative writing.

DeHaan and Havighurst divided the intellectually gifted into two groups for educational purposes. The highest 1 per cent they refer to as "first order or extremely gifted," and the remaining upper 10 per cent are the second-order gifted. They point out that the extremely gifted are very rare and probably deserve a different type of educational experience than the second-order gifted. The IQ may serve as a base instrument for the screening or pointing up of certain kinds of giftedness but at the same time, all teachers have the responsibility to attempt to determine the varieties of giftedness present in their classroom. Our plea is to use more than the IQ in the search for the gifted child.

In the past, gifted children have been more frequently found in racial groups offering superior economic, social, and educational opportunities, bat exceptions have appeared, indicating that superior abilities can occur in any of the races or ethnic groups that compose the American population. Some studics have shown that puberty is reached somewhat earlier by the gifted than by the average child. Inadequacies of gifted children generally occur in subjects requiring motor coordination.

The gifted have presented special educational problems for the public schools. Since the number of gifted is always small in comparison to the total population, it has been difficult to devise an effective system to handle them. Early solutions were to accelerate the gifted by letting them enter school early and permitting them to proceed through school at a rapid rate, with early admission both to high school and college. Some school systems have provided special schools or special classes for these exceptional children. A more common plan is to enrich the gifted child's curriculum. He is given the opportunity to go into the material of the regular classroom at greater depth; he also broadens his horizon by being forced to evaluate and determine critically his own progress and to make creative contributions and reactions to the material he is studying.

Slow-Learning Children

The slow-learning child is able to achieve extremely limited success in most school programmes, which are geared to chronological age. Slow learners proceed through the schools with a continual set of limits on their capacities. Part of this group, referred to as the educable mentally retarded and the trainable mentally retarded, require special educational facilities. The goal for these children is to provide them with some minimum standards in the area of academic skills and maximum standards in caring for self and social adjustment.

The general IQ score used to denote the educable mentally handicapped is a rating between 50 and 80. Mental maturation has been demonstrated to be a biological process which can seldom be forced through artificial means. Mentally retarded children, for instance, are rarely able to learn to read until their mental age has reached at least six years eight months to seven years. It has been demonstrated that the mentally inadequate child not only has a slower process of intellectual development, but is also limited in his abilities to absorb and cope with a variety of situations. There is a definite limitation on both the qualitative and quantitative aspects of his capacity. Mental inadequacy, then, seems generally to be a biological restriction.

CREATIVITY IN CHILDREN

Recent years have brought an increased interest in the subject of creativity. It is accepted that the traditional measures of intelligence measure at best only a few of man's abilities. If we are truly to seek out the creative child, we need to enlist a new set of measures. Torrance estimates that if we were to identify gifted children solely on the basis of intelligence tests, we would eliminate from consideration approximately 70 per cent of our most creative individuals. The difference between creativity and high scores on intelligence tests is most clearly illuminated in Torrance's findings, in which the highly creative child was differentiated on the Minnesota Tests of Creative Thinking from the highly intelligent on the Stanford-Binet. In the group studied, the highly creative ranked in the upper 20 per cent on creative thinking, but not on intelligence, while the highly intelligent group ranked in the upper 20 per cent on intelligence but not on creativity. A very small overlapping group was high on both intelligence and creativity.

It has been suggested by leaders in the field, such as Torrance, that the guidance person in the schools might well play the role of sponsoring the creative child, providing an atmosphere for communication of the child's ideas and helping to see to it that the child's creative talent is recognised. Guidance personnel can assist parents and teachers to understand the child's divergence.

The creative child is one who is daring and courageous in his thinking. He is able to break away from conformity and is open to experiences. He is ready to have one thing lead to another. This child is curious, imaginative and inventive, an innovator. Traditional intelligence tests have placed a great stress on convergent thinking, where the individual who conforms is at an advantage. The Minnesota Tests of Creative Thinking and the tests by Getzels and Jackson place less stress on the traditional academic value system and a greater stress on divergent thinking.

Guilford has spent a considerable amount of time conceptualising the creative-thinking ability and methods of assessment. The monograph by Guilford and Merrifield summarised modifications of this theory. An examination of the factors now included in Guilford's conceptual framework is of interest. Sensitivity to problems is tested, for example, by asking the subject to suggest two improvements in a common appliance. In measuring word fluency, the individual is asked to write words that end with a specified suffix or words that begin with a specified prefix. For expressional fluency, the individual is asked to write a four-word sentence when the first letter of each word is given. For word arrangement, he is required to write sentences containing four specified words. For ideational fluency, he puts down as many ideas as possible or writes as many words as possible on a given topic. Evaluation of semantic, spontaneous flexibility occurs when the individual is asked to write a variety of uses for brick or to list peculiar uses for common objects. For originality, the child is asked to write clever titles for a story or to produce symbols to represent an activity or an object. This is only a small sample of the way in which Guilford has gone about conceptualising and assessing creative thinking. However, it is apparent even from this small sample that if such tests were commonly used in the public schools we would be starting to differentiate a new type of exceptional child.

The Minnesota Tests of Creative Thinking have been divided into three categories—nonverbal tasks, verbal tasks using nonverbal stimuli, and verbal tasks using verbal stimuli. Torrance gives a detailed description of these tests.

IMPLICATIONS

1. IQ differences between boys and girls are small enough to be considered unimportant.
2. Tests do not measure some aspects of mental activity. They must be considered as samples of behaviour.
3. Grouping should not lull the teacher into believing that child study and individual needs have been taken care of through some superficial division of students.
4. A single intelligence test score does not predict a mental-growth pattern.
5. The great similarity between achievement and intelligence tests should serve as a caution when utilising these measures to study "under-achievement."
6. There are qualitative as well as quantitative differences

in intelligence.

7. Instruction should be paced to the rate of mental growth. This implies that frequent measures be taken so that some knowledge of rate is given consideration.
8. Each classroom usually includes a large range in mental and intellectual ability.
9. There is evidence of various kinds of intelligence. Any adequate inventory of "intelligence" should take into account the existence of various types, and provision should be made for involving them all in the school setting.
10. Curves based on repeated tests of individuals over time vary from curves derived from averages of mental development. Individual graphing gives a more accurate picture of intellectual development.
11. Intelligence tests do not provide absolute measures in which points between measures on the scale are equivalent. We cannot consider growth in mental age from seven to eight to represent the same distance as mental age from nine to ten.
12. Tests at different age levels measure different functions. Caution should be used in making early predictions that have long-range implications for a child's placement.
13. The culturally rich home environment frequently has a favourable influence on intelligence test scores. Children who come from "culturally deprived homes" may need additional enrichment experiences to compete equally.
14. Intelligence is also subject to fluctuations related to the child's personal-social experiences and emotional life. Great fluctuations in scores should be studied in terms of factors influencing the fluctuation. The classroom teacher should be alert to her influence on these scores.

REVIEW QUESTIONS

1. Try to secure for analysis test results of a classroom group. You might volunteer to assist a teacher with the data on his pupils, whose names could be kept confidential. Compare the range in abilities and the variance between IQ, grades, and achievement scores. What other specific data would you need to explain paradoxes that appear?
2. As you observe people about you, are you able to determine differences in their ability to do abstract, mechanical, or social tasks?? How would a view of intelligence-abstract, mechanical, and social-affect your role as a classroom teacher? How might you go about investigating mechanical and social intelligence? How would the discover" of these factors serve as an encouragement to children who may not abstract well?
3. What does Combs add to our understanding of intelligence? How does Combs differ from Thorndike, Thurstone, and Guilford? What is the difference between a psychology of possession and a psychology of use?
4. What are the implications of the nature of mental development for the instructional process? How much information regarding the mental development of a child do you feel is important for classroom planning?
5. If there is adequate evidence that the IQ is not constant at certain stages of development, what does this imply for the use of IQ's in the school? How much does a first-grade intelligence test result tell the fifth-grade teacher?
6. Discuss the significant factors which affect the possession and use of intelligence. What can teachers or parents do about these factors?
7. Formulate some specific recommendations for the promotion of intellectual development during the preschool, primary, intermediate, and junior high years. What are the respective roles of the child, parent, and teacher in these plans?
8. what are the crucial questions to ask in setting up a school testing programme to measure intelligence and achievement? Plan an elementary school testing programme to cover just these two areas. Defend your programme and the instruments selected in terms of your school's educational objectives.
9. If you can get access to individual and group scores on Intelligence tests, determine the amount of variation between the scores, and develop an explanation of the variation for these children.

10. How can the teacher get clues about the presence of mechanical, social, artistic, or creative abilities in a child without using tests?
11. If your instructor has access to individual readiness testing materials contrast these materials with group measures of readiness, and make a practical recommendation for evaluating 250 kindergarten children for first-grade readiness.

REFERENCES

A. Leahy, "Nature-Nurture and Intelligence," *Genetic Psychology* Monograph 17, 1935.

Abernethy, E., "Relationships Between Mental and Physical Growth," Monograph, Society for Research in Child Development, I, No. 7 (1936).

Anderson, J.E., "The Limitations of Infant and Pre-School Tests in the Measurement of Intelligence," *Journal of Psychology*, 8 (1939), 351-79.

Bayley, N., "Mental Growth During the First Years," *Genetic Psychology Monographs*, 14 (1933), 39.

Bayley, N., "Consistency and Variability in the Growth of Intelligence from Birth to Eighteen Years," *Journal of Genetic Psychology* (1949), pp. 165-96.

Bayley, N., "The Role of Intelligence" in *Mental Health in the Classroom*, ed. P. Witty, 13th Yearbook of the Department of Supervisors and Directors of Instruction of the National Education Association (Washington, D.C.: National Education Association, 1941), pp. 53-54.

Benda, C., "Psychopathology of Childhood" in *Manual of Child Psychology*, ed. L. Carmichael (New York: John Wiley and Sons, Inc., 1954), p. 1128.

Bloom, B., *Stability and Change in Human Characteristics* (New York: John Wiley and Sons, Inc., 1964).

Combs, A., "Intelligence from a Perceptual Point of View," *Journal of Abnormal and Social Psychology*, 47, July 1952, 662-73.

Cornell E. and C. Armstrong, "Forms of Mental Growth Patterns Revealed by Reanalysis of the Harvard Growth Data," *Child Development*, XXVI (1955), 169-204.

Courtis, S., "The Measurement of Growth,' Detroit, Mich.: 9110 Dwight Ave., 1930.

Dearborn W., and J. Rothney, *Predicting the Child's Development* (Cambridge, Mass.: Sci-Art Publishers, 1941), p. 341.

DeHaan, R., and R. Havighurst, *Educating Gifted Children* (Chicago: University of Chicago Press, 1957).

Eels, K., A. Davis, R. Havighurst, V. Herrick, and R. Tyler, *Intelligence and Cultural Differences: A Study of Cultural Learning and Problem Solving* (Chicago: University of Chicago Press, 1951).

Guilford, J.P., and P.R. Merrifield, *The Structure of Intellect Model: Its Uses and Implications*, Rep. Psychological Lab., No. 24 (Los Angels: University of Southern California, 1960).

Guilford, J.P., "Three Faces of Intellect," *American Psychologist*, 14, August 1959.

Honzik, M., "Developmental Studies of Parent-Child Resemblance in Intelligence," *Child Development*, 28 (1957) 215-28.

Inhelder, B., and J. Piaget, *The Growth of Logical Thinking from Childhood to Adolescence* (New York: Basic Books, Inc., 1958).

Kough J., and R. Dehaan, *Teacher's Guidance Handbook I, Identifying Children Who Need Help* (Chicago: Science Research Associates, 1955).

Newman, H., F.N. Freeman, and K.J. Holzinger, *1937 Twins, A Study of Heredity and Environment* (Chicago: University of Chicago Press), pp. 381-82.

Richards, T.W., "Mental Test Performance as a Reflection of the Child's Current Life Situation, A Methodological Study," *Child Development*, XXII (1951), 221-33.

Shields, J., *Monozygotic Twins: Brought up Apart and Brought up Together"* (New York: Oxford University Press, Inc., 1962).

Shuttleworth, F., "The Physical and mental Growth of Girls and Boys Age Six to Nineteen in Relation to Age at Maximum Growth," Society for Research in Child Development Monograph, 1939, 4, No. 3.

Skodak M., and H.M. Skeels, "A Final Follow-up of One Hundred Adopted Children," *Journal of Genetic Psychology*, 75 (1949), 85-125.

Spearman, C., *The Abilities of Man* (New York: The Macmillan Company, 1927).

SRA Examiner's Manual, *Primary Mental Abilities* for Grades 4-6 (Chicago: Science Research Associates, Inc., 1963), p. 5.

Terman L., and M. Merrill, *Measuring Intelligence: A Guide to the Administration of a New Revised Stanford-Binet Test of Intelligence* (Boston: Houghton Mifflin Company, 1937).

Terman, L.M., *The Measurement of Intelligence: an Explanation of and a Complete Guide for the Use of the Stanford Revision and Extension of the Binet-Simon Intelligence Scale* (Boston: Houghton Mifflin Company, 1916).

Thorndike, E.L., *The Measurement of Intelligence* (New York: Teachers College, Columbia University, 1926).

Thurstone, L.L., *The Differential Growth of Mental Abilities*, No. 14 (Chapel Hill: University of North Carolina Psychometric Laboratory, 1955).

Torrace, E.P., *Guiding Creative Talent* (Englewood Cliffs, N.J.: Prentice-Hall, Inc., 1962).

W. Olson and B. Hughes, "Subsequent Growth of Children with and without Nursery school Experience," National Society for the Study of Education, *Intelligence: Its Nature and Nurture*, 39th Yearbook, Part II (Bloomington, Ill.: Public School Publishing Co., 1940), pp. 237-44.

Wechsler, D., *The Measurement and Appraisal of Adult Intelligence* (Baltimore, Md.: Williams and Wilkins, 1958).

5

Mental Health Services: Organisation

> A man should learn to detect and watch that gleam of light which flashes across his mind from within, more than the lustre of the firmament of bards and sages. Yet he dismisses without notice his thought, because it is his. In every work of genius we recognize our own rejected thoughts: they come back to us with a certain alienated majesty.
>
> —*Ralph Waldo Emerson*

The discussion places emphasis on the tremendous growth of managed care and the attempts to gain parity in insurance. Understanding these issues can inform the decisions made by people with mental health problems and disorders, as well as their family members and advocates, and health care administrators and policymakers. Earlier chapters reviewed data on the occurrence of mental disorders in the population at large and described the treatment system. In each stage of the life cycle, issues related to mental health services have been discussed, including, for example, the breadth of mental health and human services involved in caring for children with mental health problems and disorders; deinstitutionalization and its role in shaping contemporary mental health services for children and adults; the problems associated with discontinuity of care in a fragmented service system; and the importance of primary care medical providers in meeting the mental health needs of older persons. Special mental health services concerns such as homelessness, criminalization of persons with mental illness, and disparities in access to and utilization of mental health services due to racial, cultural, and ethnic identities as well as other demographic characteristics have been discussed throughout the report.

There are four main sections in this chapter. The first section provides an overview of the current system of mental health services. It describes where people get care and how they use services. The next section presents information on the costs of care and trends in spending. The third section discusses the dynamics of insurance financing and managed care. It also addresses both positive and adverse effects of managed care on access and quality and describes efforts to guard against untoward consequences of aggressive cost-containment policies. The final section documents some of the inequities between general medical and mental health care and describes efforts to correct them through legislation, regulation, and financing changes.

The Structure of the U.S. Mental Health Service System

A broad array of services and treatments exists to help people with mental illnesses—as well as those at particular risk of developing them—to suffer less emotional pain and disability and live healthier, longer, and more productive lives. Mental disorders and mental health problems are treated by a variety of caregivers who work in diverse, relatively independent, and loosely coordinated facilities and services—both public and private—that researchers refer to, collectively, as the *de facto mental health service system* (Regier et al., 1978; Regier et al., 1993).

About 15 percent of all adults and 21 percent of U.S. children and adolescents use services in the de facto system each year. The system is usually described as having four major components or sectors:

- The *specialty mental health* sector consists of mental

health professionals such as psychiatrists, psychologists, psychiatric nurses, and psychiatric social workers who are trained specifically to treat people with mental disorders. The great bulk of specialty treatment is now provided in outpatient settings such as private office-based practices or in private or public clinics. Most acute hospital care is now provided in special psychiatric units of general hospitals or beds scattered throughout general hospitals. Private psychiatric hospitals and residential treatment centers for children and adolescents provide additional intensive care in the private sector. Public sector facilities include state/county mental hospitals and multiservice mental health facilities, which often coordinate a wide range of outpatient, intensive case management, partial hospitalization, and inpatient services. Altogether, slightly less than 6 percent of the adult population and about 8 percent of children and adolescents (ages 9 to 17) use specialty mental health services in a year.

The *general medical/primary care* sector consists of health care professionals such as general internists, pediatricians, and nurse practitioners in office-based practice, clinics, acute medical/surgical hospitals, and nursing homes. More than 6 percent of the adult U.S. population use the general medical sector for mental health care, with an average of about 4 visits per year—far lower than the average of 14 visits per year found in the specialty mental health sector. The general medical sector has long been identified as the initial point of contact for many adults with mental disorders; for some, these providers may be their only source of mental health services. However, only about 3 percent of children and adolescents contact general medical physicians for mental health services; the human services sector plays a much larger role in their care.

- The *human services* sector consists of social services, school-based counseling services, residential rehabilitation services, vocational rehabilitation, criminal justice/prison-based services, and religious professional counselors. In the early 1980s, about 3 percent of U.S. adults used mental health services from this sector. But by the early 1990s, the National Comorbidity Survey (NCS) revealed that 5 percent of adults used such services. For children, school mental health services are a major source of care (used by 16 percent), as are services in the child welfare and juvenile justice systems, which serve about 3 percent.
- The *voluntary support network* sector, which consists of self-help groups, such as 12-step programs and peer counselors, is a rapidly growing component of the mental and addictive disorder treatment system. The Epidemiologic Catchment Area (ECA) study demonstrated that about 1 percent of the adult population used self-help groups in the early 1980s; the NCS showed a rise to about 3 percent in the early 1990s.

TABLE 1

Proportion of adult population using mental/ addictive disorder services in one year

Total Health Sector	11%*
Specialty Mental Health	6%
General Medical	6%
Human Services Professionals	5%
Voluntary Support Network	3%
Any of Above Services	15%

*Subtotals do not add to total due to overlap.

Source: Regier et al., 1993; Kessler et al., 1996

TABLE 2

Proportion of child/adolescent populations (ages 9–17) using mental/addictive disorder services in one year

Total Health Sector	9%*
Specialty Mental Health	8%
General Medical	3%
Human Services Professionals	17%*
School Services	16%
Other Human Services	3%
Any of Above Services	21%

*Subtotals do not add to total due to overlap.
Source: Shaffer et al., 1996

The Public and Private Sectors

The de facto mental health service system is divided into public and private sectors. The term"public sector" refers both to services directly operated by government agencies (e.g., state and county mental hospitals) and to services financed with government resources (e.g., Medicaid, a Federal-state program for financing health care services for people who are poor and disabled, and Medicare, a Federal health insurance program primarily for older Americans and people who retire early due to disability). Publicly financed services may be provided by private organizations. The term"private sector" refers both to services directly operated by private agencies and to services financed with private resources (e.g., employer-provided insurance). Funding for the de facto mental health service system is discussed later in the report.

State and local government has been the major payer for public mental health services historically and remains so today. Since the mid-1960s, however, the role of the Federal government has increased. In addition to Medicare and Medicaid, the Federal government funds special programs for adults with serious mental illness and children with serious emotional disability. Although small in relation to state and local funding, these Federal programs provide additional resources. They include the Community Mental Health Block Grant, Community Support programs, the PATH program for people with mental illness who are homeless, the Knowledge Development and Application Program, and the Comprehensive Community Mental Health Services for Children and Their Families Program.

The fact that 16 percent of the U.S. adult population—largely the working poor—have no health insurance at all is the focus of considerable policy activity. Many others are inadequately insured. Initiatives designed to increase enrollment for selected populations include the newly created Child Health Insurance Program, which provides block grants to states for coverage of children not eligible for Medicaid.

These federally funded public sector programs buttress the traditional responsibility of state and local mental health systems and serve as the mental health service"safety net" and"catastrophic insurer" for those citizens with the most severe problems and the fewest resources in the United States. The public sector serves particularly those individuals with no health insurance, those who have insurance but no mental health coverage, and those who exhaust limited mental health benefits in their health insurance.

Each sector of the de facto mental health service system has different patterns and types of care and different patterns of funding. Within the specialty mental health sector, state- and county-funded mental health services have long served as a safety net for people unable to obtain or retain access to privately funded mental health services. The general medical sector receives a relatively greater proportion of Federal Medicaid funds, while the voluntary support network sector, staffed principally by people with mental illness and their families, is largely funded by private donations of time and money to emotionally supportive and educational groups. The relative quality of care in these various sectors is a matter of intense interest and discussion, although there is little definitive research to date.

Effective functioning of the mental health service system requires connections and coordination among many sectors (public–private, specialty–general health, health–social welfare, housing, criminal justice, and education). Without coordination, it can readily become organizationally fragmented, creating barriers to access. Adding to the system's complexity is its dependence on many streams of funding, with their sometimes competing incentives. For example, if as part of a Medicaid program reform, financial incentives lead to a reduction in admissions to psychiatric inpatient units in general hospitals and patients are sent to state mental hospitals instead, this cost containment policy conceivably could conflict with a policy directive to reduce the census of state mental hospitals.

The public and private parts of the de facto mental health system treat distinct populations with some overlap. 11 percent of the U.S. population use specialty or general medical mental health services each year. Nearly 10 percent of the population—almost all users—received some care in private facilities, while 2 percent of the population received care in public facilities. About 1 percent of the population used inpatient care; of these, one-third received care in the public sector, suggesting that those requiring more intensive services rely more heavily on the public safety net (Regier et al., 1993; Kessler et al., 1994). Nonetheless, many people with severe and persistent illness now receive at least some of their care in the private sector. This makes it important to ensure that the private sector can meet the full treatment needs of this population.

PATTERNS OF USE

Adults

Americans use the mental health service system in complex ways, or patterns. A total of about 15 percent of the U.S. adult population use mental health services in any given year. These data come from two epidemiologic surveys: the Epidemiologic Catchment Area (ECA) study of the early 1980s and the National Comorbidity Survey (NCS) of the early 1990s. Those surveys defined mental illness according to the prevailing editions of the *Diagnostic and Statistical Manual of Mental Disorders* (i.e., DSM-III and DSM-IIIR) and defined mental health services in accordance with the "de facto" system described above. A hierarchy of sectors in the treatment system (i.e., specialty mental health, general medical, and other human services). About 6 percent of the adult population use specialty mental health care; 5 percent of the population receive their mental health services from general medical and/or human services providers, and 3 to 4 percent of the population receive their mental health services from other human service professionals or self-help groups. (The overlap across these latter two sectors accounts for these figures totaling more than 15 percent).

Also, slightly more than *half* of the 15 percent of the population that use mental health services have a specific mental or addictive disorder (8 percent), while the remaining portion has a mental health problem or a disorder not included in the ECA or NCS (7 percent). The surveys estimate that during a 1-year period, about one in five American adults— or 44 million people— have diagnosable mental disorders, according to reliable, established criteria. To be more specific, 19 percent of the adult U.S. population have a mental disorder alone (in 1 year); 3 percent have both mental and addictive disorders; and 6 percent have addictive disorders alone. Consequently, about 28 percent of the population have either a mental *or* addictive disorder (Regier et al., 1993; Kessler et al., 1994).

Given that 28 percent of the population have a diagnosable mental or substance abuse disorder and only 8 percent of adults both have a diagnosable disorder and use mental health services, one can conclude that less than one-third of adults with a diagnosable mental disorder receives treatment in one year. In short, a substantial *majority* of those with specific mental disorders do not receive treatment. 28 percent of the U.S. adult population who meet full criteria for a mental or addictive disorder, and illustrates that 8 percent receive mental health services while 20 percent do *not* receive such services in a given year.

Among the service users with specific disorders, between 30 and 40 percent perceived some need for care. However, most of those with disorders who did not seek care believed their problems would go away by themselves or that they could handle them on their own (Kessler et al., 1997). In a recent 1998 Robert Wood Johnson national household telephone survey, 11 percent of the population perceived a need for mental or addictive services, with about 25 percent of these reporting difficulties in obtaining needed care (Sturm & Sherbourne, 1999). Worry about costs was listed as the highest reason for not receiving care, with 83 percent of the uninsured and 55 percent of the privately insured listing this reason. The inability to obtain an appointment soon enough because of an insufficient supply of services was listed by 59 percent of those with Medicaid but by far fewer of those with private insurance.

Children and Adolescents

Comparable data on service use by children and adolescents with diagnoses of mental disorder and at least minimal impairment only recently have been obtained from a National Institute of Mental Health (NIMH) multisite survey of children and adolescents ages 9 to 17 years (Shaffer et al., 1996).

Although 9 percent of the entire child/adolescent sample received some mental health services in the health sector (that is, the general medical sector and specialty mental health sector), the largest provider of mental health services to this population was the school system. Nearly 11 percent of the child/adolescent sample received their mental health services exclusively from the schools or the human services sector (with no services from the health sector); another 5 percent received school services in addition to health sector services. Many children served by schools do not have diagnosable mental health conditions covered in available surveys—some may have other diagnoses such as adjustment reactions or acute stress reactions. In addition, 1 percent of children and adolescents received their mental health services from human service professionals, such as those in child welfare and juvenile justice. The latter is a setting under increasing scrutiny as the result of pending Federal legislation. At present, child data are unavailable that would exactly match the adult data on service use (analyzed by diagnostic severity and by public versus private sectors).

Almost 21 percent of children and adolescents (ages 9 to 17) had some evidence of distress or impairment associated with a specific diagnosis and also had at least a minimal level of impairment on a global assessment measure. Almost half of this group (almost 10 percent of the child/adolescent population) had some treatment in one or more sectors of the de facto mental health service system, and the remainder (more than 11 percent of the population) received no treatment in any sector of the health care system. This translates to a majority with mental disorders not receiving any care. Of the 21 percent of the young population receiving any mental health services, slightly less than half (about 10 percent) met full criteria for a mental disorder diagnosis; the remainder (more than 11 percent of the population) received diagnostic or treatment services for mental health problems, conditions that do not fully meet diagnostic criteria (Shaffer et al., 1996).

In summary, the mental health treatment system is a dynamic array of services accessed by patients with different levels of disorder and severity, as well as different social and medical service needs and levels and types of insurance financing. Disparities in access due to sociocultural factors have been described in earlier sections of this report. In a system in which substantial numbers of those with even the most severe mental illness do not receive any mental health care in a year, the match between service use and service need is clearly far from perfect. Neither the number nor the proportion of people with mental health problems who need or want treatment is yet established, and many factors influence perceived need for treatment, including severity of symptoms and functional disability as well as cultural factors. But obviously not everyone with a diagnosable mental disorder perceives a need for treatment, and not all who desire treatment have a currently diagnosable disorder. Providing access to appropriate mental health services is a fundamental concern for mental health policymakers in both the public and private arenas.

REVIEW QUESTIONS

1. Write an essay on organizing and financing of mental health services.
2. Give a sketch of US Mental Health Service System.

6

Mental Retardation in India

> Iron rusts from disuse; stagnant water loses its purity and in cold weather becomes frozen; even so does inaction sap the vigors of the mind.
>
> —*Leonardo Da Vinci*

India is a vast country covering over 3.3 million square kilometres is the second largest country after China. It contains 16 per cent of the world's population and has only 2.2 per cent of its area. As per 1991 census, India's pupation is estimated at 843 .93 million, spread unevenly across 25 States and 7 Union Territories. More than 15 per cent of the population live in rural areas, while about 10 per cent of them are increasingly becoming part of a newly evolving marginal habitat-semi urban areas.

India has not conducted any national survey on the nature and magnitude of disability and impairments in the country. The Census Organisation used to collect data on physical infirmities in the decennial census during 1861 to 1941. This practice was discontinued owing to doubts regarding the reliability of such data. This practice was partially resumed in 1981. However, no information was gathered regarding prevalence of persons with mental handicaps. In the past some sample surveys have attempted to estimate the prevalence of mentally handicapped population in select areas. But, a total picture does not emerge from these surveys. Even the National Sample Survey on Disabled Persons carried out in 1981 has sadly excluded mental disability from its purview.

Any proposal for conduct of a National Survey of mental disabilities is beset with problems related to financial outlay, difficult terrain to traverse along the length and breadth of the country, multi-lingualism, paucity of trained manpower to undertake such exercises, etc. A few sample surveys have used psychometric tests and labelled approximately three per cent of the general population as "mentally retarded". This implies that the retarded population in India could be anywhere near the alarming figure of 26 million.

Role of Government

In pre-independent India, there was practically no initiative from the government to introduce any services for persons with mental handicaps. Neither, there was any demand to initiate services for these persons since public awareness on mental disabilities was dismally low. Besides, public attitudes towards mentally disabled persons oscillated ambivalently between pity, tolerance or superstition at one end to apathy or ignorance at the other.

It was against this background that in 1950, for the first time, Government of India recognised disabled persons as an equal and rightful participants in the social and economic activities of the nation. This was guaranteed by the Constitution of India before Central and State Governments began expressing concern for welfare of the disabled by initiating several programmes or schemes for these persons.

(a) Welfare Sector

On 25th September, 1985, the Central Government constituted a new Ministry of Welfare by bringing the subject of handicapped welfare under one of its five bureaus. In contemporary India, the responsibility of implementing welfare schemes for the handicapped is shared between Central as well as State governments. Broadly, the Centre is responsible for formulating welfare policies and programmes apart from coordinating, guiding or promoting implementation of welfare services by State governments.

In order to effectively deal with the multi-dimensional problems of the handicapped, the Central government established four national institutes, one in each area of disability.

The National Institute for the Mentally Handicapped (NIMH), Secunderabad, was established in 1984 as an autonomous body under Ministry of Welfare, Government of India. The NIMH is to serve as an apex organisation for manpower development, growth of suitable models of service delivery and for undertaking research in areas related to early identification, training and rehabilitation of persons with mental handicaps. The NIMH is also to serve as a premier information and documentation centre in the area of metal retardation.

Apart form the recently established NIMH, there are other national bodies in the country which are also actively engaged in research, training and service programmes for the mentally handicapped.

(i) All India Institute of Physical Medicine and Rehabilitation, Bombay;

(ii) All India Institute of Speech and Hearing, Mysore;

(iii) Government Institute of Re Madras;

(iv) The Institute for Physically Handicap;

(v) The National Institute of Rehabilitation Training and Research, Orissa;

(vi) All India Institute of Medical Sciences. New Delhi;

(vii) National Institute of Mental Health and Neurosciences. Bangalore.

The Ministry of Welfare has also set up a National Council on Handicapped Welfare to frame policy guidelines for the entire country and to determine priorities. The Government of India has special schemes for granting annual National Awards for outstanding employers of persons with mental handicap as well as employees with mental disabilities. This serves as an incentive for people to come forward and employ mentally retarded persons. Other beneficial schemes for the mentally handicapped are travel concessions in Indian Railways, Children's Educational Allowance, providing reimbursement of Rs. 50 per month to Central Government employees having children with mental handicaps. Besides, there are income-tax concessions for parents of the mentally handicapped children. Recently a comprehensive scheme for providing Community Based Rehabilitation Services (CBRS) for mentally handicapped persons hailing from rural areas has also been initiated by the Ministry.

(b) Education Sector

Some of the policies and programmes adopted by Ministry of Education. Government of India, has fringe benefits for children with mental handicap. Article 45 of the Indian Constitution emphasises that the State shall provide free and compulsory education for all children up to the age of 14. Based on the recommendations of several educational commissions set up by the Central Government form time to time, a National Education Policy (NEP) was enunciated in 1968. This policy provides the framework for educational expansion and development in the country. The salient features of NEP, which has relevance for mentally handicapped children, is its emphasises on provision for free and compulsory educational facilities, encouragement of Integrated Education Programmes (IEP), provision for basic resource facilities in selected educational institutions, promotion of integration of mentally handicapped children with normal or non-disabled children, etc.

The Ministry of Welfare introduced a scheme for Integrated Education for Disabled (IED) Children on an experimental basis in few states in 1974. Most of the benefits of this on going Scheme appears to reach only children with physical and/or sensory disabilities rather than the mentally handicapped children.

(c) Labour Sector

The Ministry of Labour, Government of India has been providing another source of succour for the disabled population in the country through some of its policies and programmes. The right to work and the right to public assistance in case of unemployment, provision for just and humane working conditions, minimum wages and ensuing decent standards of living are all severally recognised in different articles of the Constitution of India.

The overall employment scene for able bodied persons is itself at nascent stage in the country. Therefore, any discussion on creating employment opportunities for disabled persons, especially mentally disabled, is likely to pose radical questions on the very feasibility of such endeavours. However, there can be no two opinions on the need for providing work to the disabled citizens of the country especially in the view of adverse effects on the economy, wherein a tenth of the disabled population is workless and consequently their burden is to be shared by the non-disabled sections of society.

Some of the important programmes to promote employment for the disabled in the country include, reservation of jobs in public sector, creation of special employment exchanges for handicapped, establishment of vocational rehabilitation centers to train or place disabled persons, grant-in-aid assistance to voluntary organisations for training and employment for disabled persons, etc. However, most of these programmes do not seem to directly benefit individuals with mental handicap as much as those with other physical and/or sensory disabilities. About 90 per cent of the registrants are physically disabled, six per cent are blind and the remaining are speech and hearing impaired. There is hardly any scope for registration of mentally handicapped individuals.

Role of Voluntary Organisations

In India the voluntary sector continues to play a dominant and significant role in providing welfare and rehabilitation services for the disabled. A large number of voluntary agencies have emerged in several parts of the country in aid of the handicapped. Before Independence, many of these voluntary organisations thrived on small contributions from philanthropists or well wishers. This trend has changed recently as these organisations are increasingly becoming dependent upon grants from government and industrial establishments. Tax concessions granted by government to the individuals and industrial houses for their contribution towards welfare of handicapped has encouraged flow of funds into voluntary sector. Besides, some private foreign funding agencies have also been providing financial and material supports to voluntary organisations working for a welfare of the handicapped. Many voluntary agencies not only provide services, but also, act as potential pressure groups. While some voluntary organisations have the means to enlist professional assistance for carrying out their service activities, many of them suffer from problems owing to lack of funds, poor man-management technologies, absence of incisive professionalism, etc.

There are broadly two types of voluntary organisations serving the mentally handicapped in the country. They are:

(i) Those organised on humanitarian conditions by well meaning philanthropists or social activists; and,

(ii) Those which owe their origin to the parents or relatives of the mentally handicapped persons.

The motivation behind voluntarism in the area of mental handicap has also undergone considerable metamorphosis over the years in India. Most voluntary agencies started in the early independence days were raised on religious zeal and frank sentimentalism in favour of doing "good" to the "unfortunately" disabled as an "act of service to god". Even today, few voluntary agencies serve the mentally handicapped on such premises and are manned/supervised by missionaries of different religious faiths or by retired senior citizens with a fervour to spend the last days of their life for a "noble cause". Even if the emotional foundations of such voluntary agencies are commendable and qualify them to initiate services for mentally handicapped persons, to sustain quality services may require sound scientific persistance for marketing a "cause", which is lacking. Some voluntary agencies have been initiated by parents or relatives of mentally handicapped persons. At times, parents self help voluntarism has evolved as a result of their felt dissatisfaction or distrust about philanthropist activities.

The contemporary emphasis is on building awareness amongst parents of mentally handicapped so as to enable them to form their own self help groups. Parents are encouraged to register their associations or self help groups and even enlist professional support to run the service centre for their own children with mental handicaps. The initial experiments along these lines are proving to be, both, popular as well as successful with many parent organisations. Some parent self help groups have even gone to the extent of availing Group Insurance Schemes to ensure adequate economic and social security benefits for their children with mental handicaps. As on date, there are about forty parent self help groups scattered across the country.

Voluntarism in mental retardation is yet to come of age and maturity in India. The professional interactions between voluntary agencies are far from being mutually cooperative or coordinated. Each agency works in isolation so as to aggrandise their own self image than in the common endeavour to promote the cause of handicap welfare. This has led to some degree of slowness in the pace of welfare for individuals with mental handicap.

Growth of Institutions

The Home for Mentally Deficient Children, Mumbai, established by Children's Aid Society, in 1941 is claimed to be the first voluntary agency in India. In the fifties, eleven more schools were started in various parts of the country. Another sixty centres were added during the 1960's.

The NIMH has compiled a Directory of Institutions for Mentally Handicapped Persons in India (Reddy, 1988; 1989; 1992) in order to derive a comprehensive picture on the nature and distribution of available services in the country. By the year ending 1992, the Directory (and its supplements) have listed 485 institutions serving mentally handicapped persons spread over 19 states and 4 union territories. There are, still, six States and three Union Territories, which are not represented. The situation is particularly grim in the North-Eastern States, wherein services for mentally retarded persons are conspicuous by their absence.

Even wherein services are available, their pattern of distribution is far from being equitable or commensurate with the population/prevalence demands in that area. Fortunately, Government of India has recognised this unevenness in distribution of available services and is currently encouraging stimulation of services in unrepresented areas. There has been a three fold increase in the number of institutions for persons with mental handicaps compared to a baseline figure of around 150 agencies in 1980's. However, one must be cautious of the fact that a small percentage of these institutions listed on record may not even exist on ground, or maybe, planning to start services in due course of time.

The mere availability of institutional facilities for mentally handicapped persons cannot be considered as adequate unless the quality of such rendered services are also elaborated. Unfortunately, there is a lot to be desired from the quality of services rendered by some voluntary organisations.

Professionalism

Advances in the field of modern medicine has succeeded in improving the average life span of both mentally disabled as well as the non-disabled population. The decrease in infant mortality rates owing to increased awareness about pre-natal, natal and post-natal care, immunisation practices, prevention programmes, etc., has also contributed to a possible increase in incidence of the severe-profound categories of mental handicaps (cases that would have otherwise seen their natural demise).

Individuals with mental handicap require scientifically planned and well integrated services from the professionals, such as, peadiatrician, clinical psychologist, psychiatrist, special teacher, occupational therapist, speech therapist, physiotherapist, etc.

Before 1985, there were only about ten centers offering some form of Certificate/Diploma level courses for special teachers of children with mental handicaps. A present, there are over twenty centers which offer diploma level training to in service candidates/teachers from voluntary organisations. A uniform syllabi is prescribed for the teacher trainees, who take a common annual examination conducted by the NIMH, Secunderabad. The NIMH also offers a Bachelors Degree in Mental Retardation affiliated to Osmania University, Hyderabad. The objective of this course is to train a student to provide comprehensive service for mentally handicapped persons.

A recently compiled "Directory of Professionals in Mental Handicap in India" (Reddy. 1991) lists 795 professionals from 19 states in the country. Only 28 (3.52%) of them are trained till doctorate level, 25 (3.15%) are at pre-doctoral level, 156(19.63%) are at Master's level and 87 (10.94 %) are with graduate qualifications. Out of the remaining, 223 (28.05 %) are graduates with professional diplomas or certificates in mental retardation and 139(17.48%) are undergraduates with professional diplomas or certificates in mental retardation. Besides, there are also 137 (17.23 %) untrained persons listed in the Directory.

Admittedly, the names listed in the Directory cannot be, by any means, exhaustive. Nor do they reflect the actual state of affairs regarding manpower resources in mental retardation in India. There are several reasons for this suspicion. The mobility of persons working in the area of mental handicaps in India is very high. Many unemployed persons may work temporarily in the field until they secure better job opportunities elsewhere. The teacher income in an average special school setting is very low. Despite government recommendations on salaries for special teachers; in actual job situations, one has to brave the option of a lesser pay then the dangerous reality of remaining unemployed.

Research

The advancements in any field is often the direct result of increasing experiences as well as controlled scientific research. In the field of mental retardation, scientific research has always had a low priority. A peep into the history of mental retardation in India shows concerted efforts only by a handful of investigators. Often, owing to their individual competencies such individuals have succeeded incompleting certain projects on particular aspects of mental relation

Otherwise, research literature is replete with elaborations on specific medical syndromes, anecdotal reports, case histories or even frank sentimental advocacy in favour of the 'cause' of mental retardation. These observations do not amount to carping at the contributions already made in this relatively neglected field. Rather, it is the expression of an earnest desire to concert and coordinate a research policy or programmes for better understanding of a vexing reality: Mental Retardation.

Objective observation, experimentation, systematic law making and derivation of inferences on experienced phenomena is the main endeavour in any branch of Science. The acquired scientific knowledge is publicly disseminated by means of presentation in seminars, conferences, publication of books, journals, etc. Scientific research in the field of disability and impairments, especially mental retardation, is still at a nascent stage in India.

The first Indian journal in the field of mental retardation was the *Occupational Therapy Journal* later renamed as *The Journal of Rehabilitation in Asia* appeared from Bombay in 1960. With the formation of All India Association on Mental Retardation (AIAMR), Chandigarh, *The Indian Journal of Mental Retardation* appeared in 1968. Thereafter, the Federation for Welfare of the Mentally Retarded (FWMR), New Delhi, started a popular journal titled *Mental Retardation Digest* in 1970. None of these pioneering journals appear any more in the country. In fact, in the contemporary scene, there is no single journal exclusively publishing research articles on mental handicaps only. Rather, there are a few journals with generic interest on all disabilities and impairments. For example, *Disabilities and Impairments* is an interdisciplinary biannual research journal on all handicaps published from New Delhi since 1985. The Ministry of Welfare. Government of India, brings out *The Indian Journal of Disability and Rehabilitation* twice in a year since 1987. Mostly, research articles on mental retardation are currently published in discipline oriented journals, such as, *Indian Pediatrics, Indian Journal of Clinical Psychology, Indian Journal of Social Work,* etc.

Research in the field of rehabilitation sciences appear to be advancing at a rapid pace in the West as well as India. This is evidenced by the increasing number of research publications on topics related to disability and impairments. Despite these gradual developments, there has been no attempt to undertake a kind of stock taking on the quality and quantity of publications in the field of mental retardation in India.

It was the aim of the present study to compile a list of research titles for articles published on mental retardation in India; and, to study broad trends in the distribution of publications in relation to specific variables, such as, years, type of journal, areas of research, etc.

Methodology

The investigators approached every known/available information and documentation centre on social sciences (Appendix 1) for procuring old issues of journals. Each journal/ issue was searched for research articles published on any area related to disability and impairments, especially mental retardation.

The following inclusion/exclusion criteria were maintained during the literature search:

Inclusion Criteria

Any or all research titles related to the field of mental retardation published by Indian authors in Indian journals were included. Research articles bordering on indirect references to any aspect of mental retardation (such as, general morbidity studies on mental health conditions) were also included.

TABLE 1

Distribution of Top Fifteen Journal Research for the Present Bibliography

Rank order	*Name of Journal*	*Year of first publication*	*Periodicity*	*Screened*	
				Years	*Issues*
I	Indian Journal of Pediatrics	1933	Bimonthly	52-93	258
II	Indian Pediatrics	1964	Monthly	64-93	360
III	Indian Journal of Mental Petardation*	1968	Half yearly	68-82	30
IV	Indian Journal of Medical Research	1912	Monthly	54-93	480
V	The Journal of Rehabilitation in Asia*	1960	Quarterly	60-87	112
VI	Child Psychiatry Quarterly*	1968	Quarterly	68-89	88
VII	Indian Journal of Psychiatry	1959	Half yearly	65-92	56
VIII	Indian Journal of Disability and Rehabilitation	1987	Half yearly	87-92	12
IX	The Indian Journal of Social Work	1940	Quarterly	40-92	212
X	Indian Journal of Clinical Psychology	1974	Half yearly	74-92	38
XI	Indian Journal of Child Health*	1952	Monthly	52-63	144
XII	Social Welfare	1952	Monthly	57-87	372
XIII	Disabilities and Impairments	1987	Half yearly	87-92	12
XIV	Journal of Personality and Clinical Studies*	1985	Half yearly	85-92	16
XV	The Nursing Journal of India	1920	Monthly	64-92	348
	Mental Health Review	1981	Half yearly	81-91	22

*indicates Journals that have ceased publication currently.

Exclusion Criteria

Any or all research articles not related directly to the field of mental retardation, or were related to the field of mental retardation but published by foreign authors in Indian journals or by Indian authors in foreign journals were excluded. References quoting mimeographs, books, proceedings of conferences or seminars, video films, etc., were also excluded from the purview of the present search. As far as possible, cross references were avoided in view of the fact that they were at times incomplete, incorrect or even misleading.

The compiled list of references were periodically fed into a computer on specially designed bibliography software programme.

These top fifteen journals, between themselves, cover 913 out of 1095 (83.4%) research articles on mental retardation in this bibliography (Table 2). In other words, only 182 articles (16.62%) are shared by the remaining 87 journals screened for this bibliography.

In the present bibliography, 1095 (68.91%) research titles are directly related to the field of mental retardation (Table 3). The other fields covered under this bibliography are physical handicaps (N: 113; 7.11%), juvenile delinquency (N: 90; 5.66%), speech and hearing handicaps (N: 79; 4.97%), visual impairments (N; 26; 1.63%), infantile autism (N: 15; 0.95°%>. learning disabilities (N: 4; 0.24 %) and others (N: 128; 7.95%) respectively. The 'others' category includes research titles of general interest, such as, conduct disorders, seizure disorders, behaviour problems in children, etc.

Admittedly, the emphasis of present bibliography search has confined to the field of mental retardation. Based on a glossary prepared for this purpose (Table 4), an area-wise distributional analysis of the bibliography on menial retardation was carried out on seven distinctly identified areas, viz., medical, psychological, Psychoeducational, policy issues, psychosocial Downs syndrome and early intervention services.

TABLE 2

Journal-wise Distribution of Research Titles within the Area of Mental Retardation

Rank Order	*Name of Journal*	*N*	*Per cent*	*Cumulative*
I	Indian Journal of Pediatrics	215	19.63	19.63
II	Indian Pediatrics	133	12.15	31.78
III	Indian Journal of Mental Retardation	132	12.06	43.84
IV	Indian Journal of Medical Research	69	6.30	50.14
V	The Journal of Rehabilitation in Asia	51	4.66	54.80
VI	Child Psychiatry Quarterly	45	4.11	58.91
VII	Indian Journal of Psychiatry	42	3.84	62.75
VIII	Indian Journal of Disability & Rehabilitation	37	3.38	66.13
IX	The Indian Journal of Social Work	36	3.29	69.42
X	Indian Journal of Clinical Psychology	34	3.11	72.53
XI	Indian Journal of Child Health	32	2.92	75.45
XII	Social Welfare	25	2.28	77.73
XIII	Disabilities & Impairments	22	2.01	79.74
XIV	Journal of Personality & Clinical Studies	16	1.46	81.20
XV	The Nursing Journal of India	12	1.10	82.30
	Mental Health Review	12	1.10	83.40
	Others	182	16.62	100.00
	Total	*1095*		

The results of area wise distributional analysis based on the above mentioned glossary, reveals that most research on mental retardation has concentrated on medical aspects (N: 439; 40.09%), followed by focus on psychological aspects (N: 194; 17.72%). psychosocial aspects (N: 122; 11.14%), policy issues (N: 102; 9.32%), psychoeducational aspects (N: 94; 8.58%), Downs syndrome (N: 55; 5.02%), prevalence or epidemiological aspects (N: 38; 3.47%), services deliver (N:

26; 2.37%) and early intervention services (N: 25; 2.28%) respectively.

Further, intense analysis was carried out to discover the distribution of research titles in the bibliography in relation to specific topics within the broad areas of medical psychological, psychoeducational and psychosocial aspects of mental retardation.

The results indicate that mental retardation research has covered mainly topics like biochemical anamolies (N: 75; 17.08%), followed by investigations on nutritional disorders (N: 69; 15.49%) and so on. A bulk of psychological research on mental retardation has been devoted towards disagnostic assessment (N: 53; 27.32%), followed by writings on nature of mental retardation (N: 28; 14.43%) and so on. Psychoeducational research on mental retardation has studied teaching or training aspects (N: 47; 38.52%), followed by topics related to play/leisure/recreational aspects (N: 16; 13.11%) and vocational aspects (N: 14; 11.48%). Psychosocial research on mental retardation has frequently studied attitudes and others' perception (N: 33; 35.12%) followed by parent studies (N: 13; 13.83%) and articles on adjustment/adaptation problems in this population (N: 10; 10.64%).

A yearwise distribution of research titles within the field of mental retardation (Table 3) shows an initial spun in the quantity of research after the year 1965 compared to the period before. However, there appears to be a more or less stable production of research papers in the past 25 years.

Discussion

The present bibliography is a compilation of 1095 (68.99%) research titles directly related to the field of mental retardation from an overall 1587 listings in the field of disability and impairments. A cursory analysis shows that *Indian Journal of Pediatrics* ranks first with the highest number of research publications on mental retardation (N. 215; 19.63%) followed by *Indian Pediatrics* (N: 133; 12.15%), *Indian Journal of Mental Retardation* (N: 132; 12.06%) and soon (Table 2). However, this picture is quite different when the mean number of publications per issue in the top fifteen ranked journals are computed.

TABLE 3

Year-wise Distribution of Research Titles Within the Fields of Mental Retardation

Duration (In years)	*N*	*Per cart*	*Cumulative Per cent*
<1960	77	7.03	7.03
1961-1965	86	7.85	14.88
1966-1970	185	16.90	31.78
1971-1975	179	16.35	48.13
1976-1980	165	15.07	63.20
1981-1985	172	15.71	78.91
1986-1990	184	16.80	95.71
1991 +	47	4.29	100.00
Total	*1095*		

(Range: 1936-1993; 58 years; Mean: 18.44)

Owing to the long standing years of their existence and/or due to greater frequency in their periodicity of publication (Table 1), it appears that *Indian Journal of Pediatrics* and *Indian Pediatrics* have gained the top slots for their higher number of articles on mental handicaps. On the contrary, when the frequency of articles on mental retardation per issue is calculated, *Indian Journal of Mental Retardation* (N: 132; Mean: 4.4) ranks first followed by *Indian Journal of Disability and Rehabilitation* (N: 37; Mean: 3.083), *Disabilities and Impairments* (N: 16; Mean: 1.833) and so on. Further, it is to be noted that nearly 102 journals are represented in this bibliography and there are hardly any articles on mental retardation appearing in most of them. Probably there is only a token representation of one odd article in between several issues of these many journals. In the contemporary scenario, there is an urgent need to start a Journal exclusively for publications in the field of mental retardation. This need is justified because as many as five out of these top fifteen journals have ceased publishing currently.

The year-wise distribution of research titles within the field of mental retardation reveals an average of about 18.44 publications per year from 1936 to date. This average has almost doubled for the last decade, i.e., between 1981-85 (N: 172; Mean: 34.4) and 1986-90 (N: 184; Mean: 36.8). This implies that about thirty to forty research articles are currently being published on mental retardation every year in India.

The focus of research on menial retardation in India has all along been dominated by medical models. Nearly 439 articles (40.09%) from the present compilation of 1095 titles are on medical aspects of mental retardation. Apart from the several biochemical studies and nutritional studies by noteworthy project teams, others have mainly highlighted specific syndromes, annotated case reports or correlated specific medical aspects to mental retardation, etc. More significantly, research on preventive aspects and early intervention services have taken a backseat in the scenario of medical research on mental retardation in India. As regards to psychological aspects of mental retardation, research contributions have largely confined themselves to problems of diagnostic assessment (N:53:27.32%) and on definition of mental handicaps (N: 28; 14.43%). These trends in the focus of psychological research appear to be in consonance with the contemporary historical phase through which the field of mental retardation appears to be moving in India.

The current phase of diagnostic assessment and

identification of persons with mental retardation may soon pave way to more studies related to training/teaching and programme planning for individuals with mental disabilities in the oncoming decades. Another area of considerable neglect are studies on parents/ families of persons with mental handicaps. Wherein the long term objective is to use parent or family resources for the welfare and rehabilitation of mentally handicapped persons, there is likely to be a gradual shift of research interests to these areas in the oncoming years.

These trends and futuristic projections appear justified especially wherein one attempts to study the decade wise shift of priorities on research in mental retardation.

It appears that interest on medical aspects of mental retardation research was at its peak during the decades of 1960s and 1970s, with a gradual waning of such interests in the decade of 1980's. On the other hand, research on rehabilitative aspects seem to be on its ascendance in the recent times compared to hardly any such writings in the decades preceeding 1970's. It is heartening to note that increased importance is being given to topics like early intervention services, policy issues, psychoeducational training, etc.

REVIEW QUESTIONS

1. Explain the chief characteristics of mental health among adults.
2. What are anxiety disorders prevalanet among adults.
3. What is mood disorder?
4. Write a note on mental health in adulthood.

7

Mental Hygiene and Role of Councellor

Practically it is found that the emotional starvation of large numbers of children and adults represents a greater problem than does the physical malnutrition of which so much is heard. The psychologist who meets these emotionally starved individuals when they have reached such a state as to become problems in mental hygiene can readily point out for the counsellor certain evidences of such starvation.

Here, we are giving description of some main causes which reflect on the mental health of children.

Loneliness

One evidence of such emotional non-equilibrium is loneliness. This inner emptiness of life is felt by all humankind at times. For sonic, these times are rare; for most, they are more frequent than is ever admitted; and for others, this loneliness is so real as to create the dominant problem in their lives. The needs of those in this last category will be chiefly considered here, but methods which are effective for the last group can, to a greater or lesser degree, be used in meeting' the problems caused by loneliness in whatever sphere it may be found.

Loneliness appears in many guises, only one of which will be discussed here. For example, it often happens that those who are most lonely give the least impression of it. *The eyes of the counsellor must be keen, indeed, to detect as symptoms of loneliness an extratense, over-intense, highly-keyed demonstration of gaiety by the counsellor.* This overcompensating individual may be characterised as the "life of the party." These individuals frequently give of themselves to the utmost in the hope that they can thus keep others from being as lonely as they are. Frequently, also, by putting on such a show, it is possible for them to forget the ache of their own lives for a little while. Generally, happiness is quiet in its manifestations. The individual whose emotions are poised often leads the fun without being the "life of the party." Emotional poise comes to the individual who feels that his emotional investment in life are returned with interest, and 'who feels secure in his life relationships. If the "life of the party" could be seen alone one hour after the party, a misty eye which held back a tear, a look of having fought for something which wasn't there, is far more apt to characterize the face than the broad smile of the party hours.

There is a tragedy about these lives which may follow them throughout Friends of these typical "life-of-the-party" individuals feel that they are self-sufficient and never lonely or afraid hence, these friends bring only their laughter and lighter moments to the "life of the party." Never to have had a friend care enough to share a burden is never to have had a friend; and never to have had a friend with whom one felt free to share is to have lived a very lonely life.

Human, beings don't share burdens with those whom they feel have never carried them. The counsellor is wise who remembers in conferences with the individual student that the gay front with which that student faces the world is no guarantee of a gay spirit when that same student shuts the world out and sits alone when evening comes. Loneliness is essentially a state of psychic incompleteness, a state of tension which can be most effectively relieved by satisfying companionship. The guidance worker must always realize that there may be, and probably is, before him an individual who is lonely for the companionship of someone with whom a "oneness" is felt—someone with whom he shares, and who shares with him, that side of life which the world never sees. A feverish activity of any type on the part of an individual is almost as valid as a yellow caution signal saying, "Loneliness here." In school these students are apt to try to be in too many activities.

Their unexpressed motto seems to be, "Let me do everything, anything, so that I may not have to face the loneliness that is in me." Some of the finest people in student life are found in this category. These individuals lead uncentered lives. A futility overtone dominates their philosophy. Their need is for a sense of psychic unity with someone. That someone may be any individual with whom a sense of "oneness" can be established. The "breath of life" in a very real sense is just this common spiritual breathing with a friend—this sharing of the whole of daily living, not only life's happiness and triumph, but also its sadness and disappointment. Just as some blood types call for certain other blood types, and only certain blood types, before an effective transfusion and then adequate fusion can occur, even so it seems that some personalities require certain other personalities, and only certain other personalities, for the true fusion of friendship to be reached. The counsellor's tasks is not to find the necessary friend for the individual, but instead to point the way toward friendship.

Contrary to many popular approaches to human relationships, the student may be led to see that the real friends, those very few (any individual is fortunate who has one such friend) with whom a sense of psychic unity is established, are never won in mass. Such a friend is too vital for a full life for the student to leave to chance his ever having such a friendship. It should be pointed out to the student that this friend may be someone of the same or opposite sex, the same age or any different age, related or not related; but that when he finds this friend he will know it, for both of them will share, and life will no longer be lonely for either. The counsellor should stress the fact that the finding of such a friend is the easiest part of such a relationship, that if something beautiful is to be built in the way of a continuing sense of oneness, both must share unreservedly all of those phases of their lives which can in any way affect one another.

Further, as an aid to the student's own philosophy of friendship, the counsellor may develop some such thoughts on the following: In every human being there is some virtue worthy of the respect, the admiration, and the belief of a friend. Every human being needs to know that someone believes in him.

Friendship lifts us from what we are into what we may become. We try to measure up to the vision of someone who has faith in us. It is the part of a friend to hold fast to his faith in the best his friend can become, The power for progressive living is thus developed from vital human relationships. Few cases, indeed, would ever need the therapeutic aid of the mental hygienist if, through high school and on, every individual faced life secure in the relationship of a strong psychic unity with someone. It is the counsellor's part, first, to recognize the loneliness of these individuals who have not attained such relationships; second, to show them how to be and to hold friends; and third, to give to each individual a philosophy of friendship which will help him, when once a friend is found, to seek to understand rather than to change, to believe always the best and to be loyal.

Basic physiological trends, psychological predispositions, or other factors such as fame, fortune, beauty, and power cannot form a sufficient barrier to keep loneliness away. It is most apt to be found with the most favoured; those who walk the peaks of life are those who walk alone. The masses may bow in homage, but those who could be friends stay away because they feel they are not needed. Particularly with brilliant students the counsellor should be on the watch for loneliness. Its symptoms vary with the individual and with different individuals at different times. Though some of the most glaring symptoms can readily be recognized, it is very probably true that the counsellor must have a sense of "oneness" with the individual being counseled before the signals of loneliness which most individuals try to hide can be discerned.

The lives most people live behind their faces are lonely lives. Civilisation has brought much of comfort, but human beings at this stage of our culture are afraid of the happiness they can bring to one another. Some are so afraid of the pain which comes when a psychic tie is broken that they lack the courage ever to establish such a tie. Much stress is being placed on loneliness as a contributory cause to emotional starvation because there is so much of loneliness. Much stress is being placed on the type of human relationship which will banish this loneliness, because such relationships are rare. Yet for every human being who is capable of loneliness, and exactly to the extent that he is capable of being lonely, there is the possibility of realising this satisfying relationship. The courageous spirits who have attained great friendships have recognised that they come only through sacrifice, that there is no such thing as their springing into full bloom and continuing to be a real vital force without much of self-giving I and sharing on the part of both individuals. To those who are lonely, and that means to most human beings, the counsellor has given a great gift if he inspires them to go and find a real friend, and then to be one.

Insecurity

Insecurity is the second factor basic to much emotional starvation. When the counsellor comes to deal with the insecure student, a bit of introspection is in order. The counsellor is more humble and more able to meet the student's need if he looks within his own life and remembers how he felt when he first faced that baffling problem of inadequate expression which is at the core of insecurity. It is important that the counsellor be able to approach every counseling situation with the spirit of a helper, and not with that of a master. Especially is this true when the counseling situation involves an insecure individual.

Edward Carpenter recognised the need for such counsellor humility when he wrote:

> Who are you who go about to save them that are lost?
>
> Are you saved yourself?
>
> Do you know that who would save his own life must lose it?
>
> Are you then one of the lost?
>
> Be sure, very sure, that each of these can teach you as much as,
>
> Probably more than, you can teach them.
>
> Have you sat humbly at their feet, and waited on their lips that they
>
> Should be the first to speak—and been reverent before these
>
> children Whom you so little understand?
>
> Have you dropped into the bottomless pit from between yourself and them
>
> All hallucination of superiority, all flatulence of knowledge, and
>
> Every shred of abhorrence and loathing?
>
> Is it equal, is it free as the wind between you?

> Could you be happy receiving favours from one of the most despised of these?
>
> Could you yourself be one of the lost?
>
> Arise, then, and become a Saviour.

If there is an individual who has never known a sense of insecurity, let that individual seek his life's work elsewhere than in the counsellor's seat. One criterion for maturity is the capacity to suffer, and one of humankind's most common sufferings is an "emotional state of not being sure."

It is the mature individual who knows how to *remember* who should sit on the counsellor's side of the desk and give advice.

Very few individuals will say to a counsellor, "I brings to you this my problem of insecurity." It is the counsellor who must see what the basic problem really is, while the individual talks of troublesome surface matters which are the outgrowth of more basic causes. The counsellor's eyes must be very keen and very alert for symptoms of insecurity. These symptoms are of many kinds. For example, physical expressions of insecurity are evidenced frequently by the individual who can't find just where to put his hands, whose throat seems constantly to need to be cleared, whose color changes easily with no apparent reason—indeed, the individual whose nervous reactions are such as to focus the attention of those who are with him upon his person rather than upon his thinking. Imagination and kindness are the greatest needs of the counsellor when he is dealing with individuals dominated by a sense of insecurity.

Here, kindness can very well be born of a memory of having also suffered; for if one has lived intently and with courage and vision, there is almost surely the very real memory of the day when hands seemed made to sit on, and the chief reason for having feet seemed to be to find a place to hide them—the day when one wasn't if able to find quite the fitting words as adequate vehicles for thoughts. The counsellor's imagination might well have as its basis a knowledge of the broad psychological causes of insecurity plus a store of tact laid by through years of experience in dealing with humankind and their problems.

Most individuals feel insecure because of improper grooming. We sometimes find here the boy whose legs have outgrown his pants, and whose arms have outgrown his sleeves. For example, a boy who was giving definite trouble as an *attention-getter* in his classes was found to be wearing shirts he had outgrown. His school history until this time had been exemplary; his I.Q. was 150. Investigation showed that he was being reared by an aunt with very rigid ideas about economy. She had sent the boy to town to buy some shirts the summer before. The boy had found a shirt bargain sale, and hoping to please her had bought twelve shirts at once. The shirts were not returnable. The aunt failed to see the boy's attempt at economy by buying bargain shirts in quantity; instead, she saw the extravagance of buying more shirts than necessary. Therefore, in order to teach him a lesson, she had decreed that he must wear the shirts until he had worn them out—regardless of whether or not he had outgrown them. Four inches of his bare arm extended below the shirt cuff had proved too much for classmates at an age when teasing is one of the reasons for living, and the boy's classmates hadn't spared him. In fact, because he made better grades than any of them, they teased him with added zeal. The result was an effort on the boy's part to compensate for the felt physical insecurity by seeking attention in every other possible way. Now his father was a *very* able professional man. The difficulty was explained to the father in confidence and without his knowledge. The week following the conference with the father, the boy came to school wearing shirts that fitted him.

All insecurity problems arising from socially inadequate

clothing are not so readily solved. Frequently the individual in question is wearing hand-me-downs and has little or no money with which to buy other clothes. In such instances, conferences on making the most out of the clothes one has can be very helpful. Once the counsellor has sufficiently got the confidence of the student so that the problem can be faced, much can be done in the way of sound advice as to color combinations, possible alterations, frequent home washings and pressings, and, perhaps, in some instances a freshening by tinting. It is good technique for the individuals trying to face socially inadequate clothing problems to report to the counsellor regularly for a period of a month or so for recommendations and suggestions. In this way, the counsellor can note the actual results of the counseling which has gone before.

Improper grooming which is due to carelessness and indifference should, of course, be dealt with in a very different and in a very factual manner. The counsellor should, however, make very sure that a seeming attitude of carelessness or indifference is not a mask for lack of funds for clothes or lack of knowledge about what to wear and when to wear it. If, however, no lack of funds exists, and adequate knowledge regarding what to wear and when to wear it is found to be one of the individual's assets, the counsellor is confronted with a problem which may have such deep psychological implications that a psychologist should be brought into the case.

The counsellor's first question may be, "What motives are basic to this individual's emotional life?" Unless the breakdown of the motives which underlie these emotional strivings is complete and is faced, carelessness and indifference is apt to manifest itself, not only in clothing, but also in speech, cleanliness, manners, and habits of all kinds, studious and otherwise. Hence, the counsellor's problem is to study such an individual with reference to his emotional background.

If, after a careful examination, the counsellor finds no excuse for the manifest carelessness and indifference, the services of a trained psychologist should immediately be enlisted. However, many "clothing-indifference" problems can be handled effectively by the counsellor.

Factors Responsible for Insecurity

1. Inadequate Social Knowledge

The great prevalence of social insecurity even among adults is amply attested to by the large sale of books which deal with proper social usage. A helpful part of every alert counsellor's programme is some type of "manners club" in which proper etiquette and correct social form are both studied and practiced. Most counsellors are familiar with the girl who is socially insecure—who doesn't know when to stand up to acknowledge an introduction, when and how to take a boy's arm, or what to do at a dance when she finds herself alone—and with the boy who isn't quite sure of the proper form for introducing his new girl to his old friends, who doesn't know how to address a gentleman older than himself. When inadequate social knowledge is causing embarrassment and consequent insecurity, the counsellor's remedy is plainly adequate social knowledge.

One of the least painful ways of obtaining this knowledge is through some type of manners club. However, if such a club is to be a success, the counsellor must be very careful in the organisational approach to make sure that there is some type of social approval placed upon obtaining membership in the club. In other words, such a club is doomed to failure before it is begun if those who are members are thought to obtain membership because they have no manners or social graces. One counsellor whose manners club was quite the proper high-school club made membership obtainable only when some special school service had been performed which was considered by the counsellor, the dean, and one teacher to have sufficient worth to merit for the performer a membership in the club. In this way the counsellor was able to give the individual security by giving him a school task of responsibility which he was able to do with satisfaction to himself, and, also, those individuals who gave evidence of needing such a club were thus indirectly guided to it.

Again, social insecurity is caused by many factors other than lack of social knowledge and training. It may be that racial (or caste) distinction, occupational family background, homes on the wrong side of the tracks, divorced parents, parents in jail or otherwise without social approval, or perhaps a knowledge of illegitimacy is contributing to a person's continued sense of social insecurity. For these cases the counsellor needs to give the individual a broader sense of life's values. There is here a definite need for a reading course which will contribute toward a reorientation of personal values. The counsellor needs at hand a list of books so classified that as soon as the problem is recognized, the individual may be guided to the proper reading material.

Nor does the counsellor's task end with having given a reading-material suggestion. The counsellor-teacher relationship then comes into play, perhaps in this manner. The teacher may be sent a note suggesting that the student would like to make his next "book report" on the book the counsellor has suggested, or the public-speaking teacher may cooperate with the counsellor by asking the boy to make a speech on the subject material contained in the book. The avenues for such co-operation are legion. The counsellor's second step, however, is definite: a follow-up conference to make sure that the new and suggested values have become an active part of the individual's daily motivation; and, hence, that the social insecurity caused by the displaced value is no more.

2. Bodily Defects

Bodily defects upon which the individual is placing too much emphasis give rise to another source of physical insecurity. These defects may range all the way from pimples on the adolescent's face to a hunchback or a harelip; from a small birthmark on the forehead to a short leg or paralysed arm. These defects may, indeed, be any physical handicap over which the individual has no known control. Inasmuch as these conditions are permanent, the feelings of insecurity occasioned by them readily give way to attitudes of inferiority. No attempt is made here to summarize all the factors in life which may give rise to feelings of physical insecurity. The emphasis here is upon the need for seeking the cause of the insecurity and for helping the individual to help himself so completely that poise and personal control become dominant in that area of his life which was formerly characterised by a sense of insecurity.

3. Emotional Insecurity

The individual who is a stranger in a group and is not sure of being either wanted or accepted; the person who is dominated by the fear that he will not be liked by his fellows and who, therefore, feels conscious of himself and socially out of place when in a group; the individual who is always afraid of saying or doing the wrong thing—such individuals are emotionally insecure. Such feelings of insecurity have flowered many a party wall, and have caused tears to soak many a pillow after the party. The psychologically trained counsellor in seeking the causes of insecurity during the adolescent period should remember, while emotion is present throughout life, it is frequently strongest in its manifestations during the turbulent period of adolescence.

Emotion may be exhibited in any number of types of responses or in any combination of such responses. In terms of current psychological research, *emotion* manifests itself chiefly in adient or avoidance responses or in some degree of combination of the two. For example, love is considered as an adient response, fear and anger as avoidance responses. The teacher or counsellor, then, recognising the strong current of emotion, can hold broadly that many emotional states are derived directly from the emotional responses of *love, fear,* and *anger,* or from some combination thereof, and that emotional insecurity is almost always based upon uncertainty regarding proper outlets for the physiological tensions basic to these dominant emotions. For example, the counsellor may find himself confronted with an individual whose emotional insecurity springs from a repressed or otherwise unexpressed love emotion or, perhaps, from an unrequited love. It is possibly one of life's most desolate moments when the fact must be faced that one loves someone who doesn't love in return.

Grave doubts as to one's own worth are at once engendered. These doubts spread throughout the whole of the individual's life relationships. A general state of emotional insecurity results. Physiologically this state is, perhaps, best described as one of unrelieved tension, the extent of the emotion being determined by the intensity of the tension. Whether the counsellor gives advice to the lovelorn, or shows the individual how to effect an emotional transfer either to creative work or to some more responsive individual, depends entirely on the case. Such problems are so very frequent at the secondary-school level that the account of an experience of one of the authors may be helpful.

Emotional insecurity may just as easily be based on fear which the individual doesn't know how to face. For example, it is not uncommon for adolescents to have doubts regarding their parentage, or to be concerned lest they have cancer or some other hidden and malignant disease. Also, success has been heralded with such fervor by parents, teachers, friends, and leaders that one of the most frequently met fears is the fear of failure. Success has been talked about so much more than failure that the adolescent who finds even a normal percentage of failure in his life sometimes conies to believe himself worthless. Little does he realize that father at the dinner table tells only the success stories of his day, and that mother really does remember only the success stories of her adolescent years.

So much talk of success makes the adolescent feel unique as he honestly faces the fact that his life has more of failure in it than of success. Perhaps he worked for and hoped for the position of captain of the baseball team and in the final line-up found himself a substitute catcher. Perhaps he wanted to be president of the high-school debating team and actually found himself with no office and with the insignificant post of alternate speaker on the negative side of a question when his beliefs were entirely in sympathy with the affirmative. Perhaps he were his best Sunday blue serge suit with the long, grown-up trousers to school in the hope of getting a certain girl to consent to go to the high-school dance with him, only to find that she was going with a boy whom he very much disliked.

Teachers, parents, adolescent leaders, somehow fail to emphasize as much the many things they have dreamed about and worked for that never happened as they emphasize those few occasions in their lives when they have had the mountain-top experience of being able to say, "I wanted this, I worked for it, and I got it. I have succeeded." This problem is by no means isolated or simple. Youth is being cheated out of much of happiness and self-understanding through the "I-am-a-success" declaring habit of those to whom he turns for leadership. Consequently, the youth often enters the tasks of his life with the profound belief that he fails more frequently than does anyone else. Unless he is very sound emotionally, he is even likely to come to feel sorry for himself and thus start the groundwork for an ineffectual life.

He needs to see the uncolored facts of success and failure as they actually are in the lives of those he admires and strives to be like unto.

Continued experience of emotional insecurity based on fear readily leads to the habit of fear. The habit of being afraid has caused many individuals to go to the mental hygienist who would never have gone had the habit of fearlessness been acquired instead. One tragedy of these fear-filled lives is that this habit is sometimes inspired by the too great caution of a devoted parent. Once the habit of fear is acquired, it grows and spreads like a parasitic vine through the many and various life reactions of the individual. To be afraid one can't is the first step toward believing one can't, and believing one can't is the first step toward not being able to.

The counsellor will meet this primal emotion of fear in many, many forms. One student will confess he is afraid of failing his algebra; another that he is afraid he won't make his track letter; and another that she is afraid her boy friend loves another girl; and perhaps a fourth that she is afraid she will never be attractive. Whenever and where-ever fear presents itself, the guide's part is to inspire self-confidence. Fear grows like a gnawing pain, and rapidly; but self-confidence based on individual achievement worthy of that confidence grows even more rapidly, and as a positive force gradually wipes out the negative force of fear. The counsellor should be led to try first those things in which success is probable, and then gradually, as his confidence grows, tasks in which success is less sure. He should be taught to recognize that a step is made toward emotional adulthood when there is meaning for him in the statement that "All endeavor involves the risk of failure as well as the possibility of success."

Any situation for which the individual has no adequate patterns of reaction is likely to be a fear-producing situation.

There is no fear known to man which may not be dominating the adolescent and causing within him a high degree of emotional insecurity. Fear is an elemental emotion. The alert counsellor is ever on the watch for its manifestation. Anger, perhaps arising from a general feeling of injustice, frequently leads the adolescent, or any individual for that matter, into a state of emotional insecurity.

Individuals whose almost certain reactions to life's situations are negative ones; individuals who are not able to accept at face value the faith and love which comes into their lives because they can't help feeling that there must be a catch somewhere; individuals who are quick to show indifference, quick to hurt someone who loves them Jest the one who loves them should get to be the first to be indifferent or to hurt—these individuals frequently have suffered from some actual injustice somewhere in their lives, some injustice which hurt them so deeply as to color their entire life reactions. Such persons are often twelve-cylinder people in native endowment and one-cylinder persons in life expression. A part of the counsellor's job is to find them and to help them before it is too late.

The three emotional horsemen of the apocalypse are certainly unfulfilled love, fear, and anger, or some combination of these. Physiologically and psychologically these foes of emotional well-being and healthful living depress and incapacitate the individual. If these states are not recognised and dealt with, an emotionally insecure and hence handicapped individual is an almost certain result. All the handicapped are not on crutches; many of them live under the shadow of the fear in their hearts; not all of them are blind, for many of them with anger see life only through the blackness of some early injustice. Indeed, all of the handicapped are not the deaf and dumb, for many of them carry the sorrow of loving but not being loved, with the attendant depressing conviction that as individuals they are so inferior that no one can love them. In any of these states the counsellor's technique is to find the primary emotion which is failing to find adequate expression, and then, as far as possible, to lead the individual, first, to understand the cause of his own insecurity, and then to take positive steps to remedy it.

4. Economic Insecurity

Many counsellors who deal with economic insecurity feel that they are performing a socially useful service when they teach the individual to place his values elsewhere than in the economic sphere. Such a service is not enough. The primal needs requisite to survival are involved. The individual feels that he has asked for bread and been given a stone when he has asked for a path to lead him toward economic security and has been told that he should place his values elsewhere—that many phases of life are of more importance than its economic phases. Quite rightly, the individual gives first place to the impelling thought, "I want to know I can cat tomorrow and sleep tonight." This acute economic need is not generally met until the youth has finished secondary school, but economic insecurity frequently is felt intensely by the secondary-school student because of his home situation and because of the responsibilities which he knows he must face as soon as his secondary schooling is over.

The wise counsellor doesn't try to paint a rose-colored picture, nor is there any endeavor to brush away the youth's fears; instead, the energy which is going into the production of fear is directed toward constructive channels. The youth is given, as nearly as the counsellor is able to give it, a factual picture of the economic situation. His enthusiasm and imagination are enlisted in an effort to work wholeheartedly with the counsellor in an endeavor to determine in what way his own peculiar and particular abilities can most effectively be utilised in this current, not too inviting, economic order.

Thus, in a very healthy and positive manner, the youth is led to work harder and more purposefully toward a life goal which includes an occupational area for which his capacities lit him. It is the guidance worker's aim to see to it that the student loses his sense of economic insecurity in a constructive urge to develop fully his own potentialities, ever cognizant of the fact that life gives no guarantees, but that the race is frequently for the one who is prepared, for the one who knows his strength and how, and when, and where to use it.

5. Mental Insecurity

A form of insecurity which is rather infrequently encountered is mental insecurity. Perhaps the reason for the infrequency is that good minds are scarce, and generally the self-critical minds are the good minds. Morons make with dogmatic certainty statements that would cause the genius to ponder long. Frequently, because of thorough thinking processes, possessors of good minds remain silent while glib lesser minds influence the day. However, the evaluation of the multitude often becomes the evaluation that these individuals accept for themselves if thus far in life their mental efforts have brought them little of the fruits of success. After a few occasions of seeing the smooth-of-tongue gain the day, these individuals are very likely to feel not too certain of their own merits and accept the status given them by the multitude. When these timid minds do gather courage to express themselves, they often recognize the many qualifications necessary for any factual statement to be made, and are likely to speak with such *uncertainty* that those who hear catch only the doubt and not the thought. Soon these individuals conic to feel the need of supporting authority from other minds. Instead of bodily speaking out in the dignity of their own right as breathing, effecting, and thinking human beings, they cast about for the thoughts of someone else which are similar to their own in the hope that the authority of an accepted name will win acceptance for the thought contribution. And thus, instead of walking fearlessly and alone, they begin to walk fearfully and on mental crutches.

Unless these individuals are found and guided adequately in school, their sense of mental insecurity will very probably relegate their good minds to places of mediocrity in life. They suffer from too great respect for others and from too little respect for themselves. The wise counsellor who knows the intelligence scores of those who are counseled will be on guard for this type of insecurity among brilliant students. When it is found, the counsellor must lead the student to see the difficulty within himself and then to recognize his own value. These individuals are among the few who are sometimes benefited by knowing their I.Q. scores. Mental insecurity caused by real inferiority is sometimes found in the too bold and often exponentially limited individuals who make statements for *effect*, in the overly dramatic persons whose distrust of the validity of their own knowledge is such that they seek to hold the center of attention by an overpowering emotional appeal.

Summing Up

Loneliness and insecurity are two great contributors toward emotional starvation. The counsellor who helps students to meet and defeat these two heralds of misery' has functioned effectively in one very important sphere of counseling opportunities.

Mental hygiene is a basic ground on which the edifice of a student's personality is devised and constructed. Loneliness and insecurity are the two prime factors causing disturbance to mental hygiene and consequently on the mental health. A good counsellor (who may be a teacher or a professional) can play great role in maintaining or retaining the sound mental health of children.

REVIEW QUESTIONS

1. What do you understand by 'mental hygiene' and 'mental health'?
2. Describe a counsellor's role in maintaining sound mental health of children.
3. What are the prime factors influencing mental hygiene of children?
4. What is 'loneliness'? Suggest ways to overcome the problem.
5. What is 'insecurity'? Describe various types of the problem. Gather inferences from your surrounding and make case history.

REFERENCES

Carpenter Edward (1955), *Towards Democracy*, A. and C. Boni, New York).

Elliot and Elliot (1936), *Solving Personal Problems*, Henry Holt and Co., New York.

8

Forgetting

Life cannot go on without much foregetting

—Honore De Balzac

The career of a great man remains an enduring monument of human energy. The man dies and disappears, but his thoughts and acts survive, and leave an indelible stamp upon his race.

—Samuel Smiles, Character

'Forgetting' refers to the apparent loss of information already encoded and stored in Long term memory. Much is forgotten but enough endures so that we have a sketchy record of our lives.

Much of what we think we have forgotten does not really qualify as 'forgotten' because it was never encoded and stored in the first place. Some information, due to lack of attention may not have reached Short term memory from the sensory register; or due to inadequate encoding and rehearsal, the information may not have been transferred from Short term memory to Long term memory.

Constructive processes at work during the process of encoding distort what is stored in memory and we remember the distortions. For instance, we remember the gist or meaning,

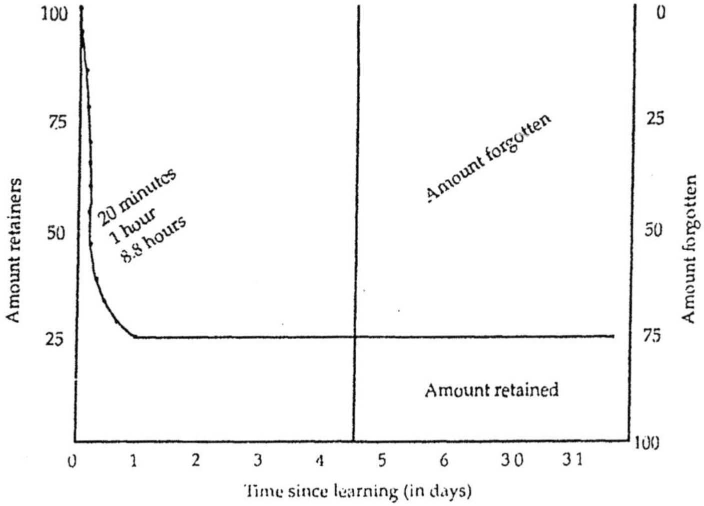

Figure 1

of what we have heard in a conversation but not the actual words themselves; we remember inferences constructed at the time the information was encoded for storage; or we encode only portions of the to-be remembered information. Strictly speaking, such faulty remembering is not forgetting. In fact, we remember what is stored we think we forgot because what we remember is not an accurate representation of what really happened.

Causes of Forgetting

Interference: can take two forms, the retroactive interference, information currently being learned interferes with information already present in memory. If learning the rules of a new board game causes you to forget the rules of a similar game you learned to play last year, you are a victim of retroactive interference. Proactive interference, in contrast, occurs when previously learned information interferes with information you are acquiring at present. If information you acquired about operating an old VCR interferes with your ability to operate a new one that has very different control, you are experiencing the impact of proactive interference.

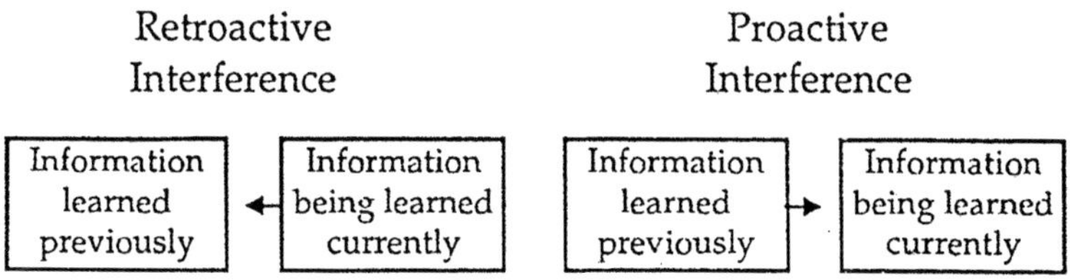

The trace decay hypothesis: Forgetting with the passage of time : perhaps the simplest view of forgetting is that information entered into long term memory fades or decays with the passage of time. This suggestion is consistent with our informal experience: Often, information we acquired quite sometime ago is more difficult to remember than information learned only recently. Yet considerable evidence suggests that this is probably not the key mechanism in forgetting.

Let us consider a classic study conducted by Jenkins and Dallenbach (1924) the researchers asked two participants to learn a list of ten nonsense syllables. In one condition, both individuals then went directly to sleep. In another, they continued with their normal activities. The participants recall of the nonsense syllables was tested after one two, four or eight hours. Results indicated that forgetting was more rapid when the individuals stayed awake than when they went to sleep. These findings argue against the suggestion that forgetting is largely the result of gradual decay of information over time.

Unfortunately, there are several problems with this study. Participants who went to sleep learned the nonsense syllables in the evening. Those who remained awake learned them in the working. Obviously, differences in circadian rhythms may have played a role in the obtained results. And indeed, sleep during the day does not seem to reduce forgetting as reported by Jenkins and Dallenbach.

However, other research in which animal subjects have been kept awake but prevented from moving about and engaging in normal activities, also indicates that forgetting is not merely a matter of the passage of time. In one such study, for example, Minami and Dallenbach (1946) taught cockroaches to avoid a dark compartment by giving them an electric shock whenever they entered it. After they had mastered this simple task, subjects were either retained in a paper cone or permitted to wander around a darkened cages at will. Results again argued against the trace decay hypothesis: subjects permitted to move about showed substantially more forgetting over a given period of time.

Retrieval problems: Without appropriate retrieval cues the sought for items stored in long term memory may not be found - one 'forgets. But while we often cannot recall something while actively searching for it, we may later recall the sought for information when we have given up the search and are doing something else. The new activity in which we are engaged, or the new context, gives us another set of appropriate reminders, or retrieval cues. And perhaps the new situation leads us to search through portions of long term memory store not examined before. The result is that we suddenly remember what we could not previously retrieve.

Thus when we think we have forgotten something, it is often a good idea to give up and do something else in order to generate new retrieval cues. Also reconstructive processes present at the time of retrieval can act to distort our recall of what is stored in our long term memory. We may remember something that did not happen and forget what did happen.

Emotional factors can also play a role in the retrieval failure that is the cause of so much forgetting. State dependent memory is an example. If we encode information while in one emotional state and try to retrieve it in another, our recall may suffer. Another more common and powerful hindering influence of emotions on retrieval is found in the phenomenon of forgetting - difficulties with the retrieval of unpleasant, anxiety - provoking information stored in long term memory.

Motivated forgetting: Many lapses of memory in daily life illustrate motivated forgetting. For example, because a man does not like meat, He may forget that his wife asked him to buy some meat for dinner. One may forget the names of people one does not like. But Freud went further than such direct, common sense examples. In the "Psychopathology of Everyday life"; Freud charmingly analyses his own memory lapses to illustrate the forgetting of such associations. He forgets a conversation he had with a man he disliked, he forgets the location of a searched for shop because he had an argument with a family that lived in the building where the shop was located; he forgets names, not because they themselves provoke displeasure but because they are associated in someway with anxiety provoking ideas; and so on through a wide range of retrieval failures.

Retrieval of the forgotten material eventually occurred. But according to psychoanalysis, some stored information is so threatening and anxiety arousing that its retrieval is possible only under special circumstances. Thus some emotionally toned information becomes available for conscious thought it is said to be in unconscious. To dredge up unconscious, repressed memories, psychoanalysts use the method of free-association-having an individual say whatever comes to the mind. Hypnosis and various drugs are also used to retrieve repressed information not available to consciousness in the normal waking state.

Amnesia

It is a profound memory deficit due either to the loss of what has been stored or to the inability to form new memories. Some amnesias have a biological basis; the memory machine - the brain is disturbed in some way. These may be called biological amnesias. The other is psychological, without any known brain malfunction, these amnesias result from major disturbances in the processes of information encoding, storage and retrieval.

(a) Psychological amnesia: when we think of amnesia, we often have in mind the person who forgets almost everything including his or her identity. But in a sense, everyone is an amnesia victim; we remember very little of our early childhoods and our dreams.

(b) Childhood amnesia: Both formal studies and common experience agree on the poverty of early memory why is our

early childhood memory so poor? Sigmund Freud (1938) used the 'repression' concept to account for childhood amnesia. He said that we are unable to retrieve childhood memories because they are associated with the forbidden, guilt-arousing, sexual and aggressive urges, he thought characterised early childhood. These urges and their associations are repressed and cannot be retrieved. They are forgotten - because being aware of them would result in strong feelings of guilt or anxiety. Another interpretation of childhood amnesia stresses differences in the ways young children and older people encode and store information. As adults, much of our memory is encoded verbally and tied into networks or schema that are based on language; it is probably no accident that language development and the richness of memory go hand in hand. But when we were very young and without language, we encoded memories in a non-verbal form, perhaps storing information as images or feelings. Early childhood memories are thus said to be stored in forms no longer available to us as verbal adults, our language dominated memories do not have retrieval cues appropriate for gaining access to the image and feeling memories of early childhood.

One more interpretation of childhood amnesia is that it may not be very 'psychological' at all. The brain is maturing and growing in the first few y;ears after birth. Perhaps the memory machine is just not able to store long term memories until the maturation is essentially finished language ability and memory develop together according to this interpretation, because both depend on brain maturation.

(c) Biological Amnesia: Concussions (brain bruises) from blows on the head, other damage to brain, temporary disturbances in the brain blood supply, certain drugs and brain diseases are some of the major biological causes of amnesia.

(d) Dream Amnesia: We dream several times each night but we remember few of these experiences. Freud's (1900-1953) interpretation of dreams was based, as was his interpretation of childhood amnesia, on repression. He considered dreams to be expressions of forbidden sexual or aggressive urges. These urges can produce strong guilt or anxiety if we become aware of them in ourselves. So their expression in dreams is hidden behind a disguise - the actual content of a dream. But even the disguised urges - dreams - have the capacity to generate some guilt or anxiety feelings. Hence they are forgotten.

Other interpretations stress the differences in the symbol systems used in dreaming and waking. If the memory symbol networks of waking life are different from those of dreaming, we may have difficulty retrieving dreams in the waking state.

The dreaming brain seems to be in a special state different from that of the working brain. Thus dream amnesia may be just another example of state dependent memory.

(e) Transient Global Amnesia: This is a profound memory problem with no loss of consciousness. It comes on suddenly without any obvious cause and it typically lasts for only a few hours or days before memory becomes normal again. Fortunately, most people who experience such amnesia have it only once. This type of amnesia is called *'global'* because so much of what has already been stored in memory is forgotten and because, even though the victim is conscious and can go about the routine business of daily life, new memories are formed while the attack is in progress. In other words, both retrograde amnesia (forgetting events one was exposed to in the past) and anterograde amnesia (the inability to encode and store new information) characterize transient global amnesia. The cause of transient global amnesia is not known, but a currently favoured hypothesis is that it is due to temporary alterations in the normal pattern of blood flow to the brain.

(f) Defensive Amnesia: People with this form of amnesia may forget their names, where they have come from, who their spouses are and many other important details of their past lives. It is called defensive because this type of amnesia is usually considered to be a way of protecting oneself from the guilt or anxiety that can result from intense, intolerable life situations and conflicts. We often wish we could forget a nagging problem. Defensive amnesia is thus an extreme form of repression.

(g) Diseases of the Brain: Among the diseases that can result in amnesia are syphilis of the brain and other brain infections, strokes and other permanent disorders of the brain blood flow brain tumours, disorders of brain metabolism, multiple sclerosis, various conditions caused by toxic chemicals, senile dementia, and primary degenerative dementia.

(h) Marijuana, Alcohol and Amnesia: Marijuana appears to have a limited short-lived effect on the encoding, storage and retrieval of information, but it can hardly be said to result in amnesia. Even when marijuan is taken in relatively high doses, its memory effects fall far short of those of the most popular mind-altering drug-ethyl alcohol. After a night of heavy drinking - a high dose of alcohol - a person may have amnesia for the events that occurred while he or she was '*smashed*. When sober again, the individual's memory of events before over indulging is intact, but there is memory gap for the period of drunkenness.

A person may have amnesia for the events occurring while under the influence of alcohol because encoding and storage processes have been disrupted by the effects of the alcohol on the brain. Another theory is that information may have been stored while in the drunken state in a form not available for retrieval in the sober state. Thus alcohol - induced amnesia may be an example of state-dependent memory.

Heavy drinking over a period of years, however can result, through vitamin B deficits and other chemical imbalances in irreversible brain damage and a pattern of symptoms known as the '*Korsakoff syndrome*'. Anterograde amnesia (the inability to form new memories) is one of the prominent symptoms of this syndrome. Korsakoff patients also have some loss of what are called remote memories - remembrance of events that occurred early in their lives and memory is not the only information - processing problem of Korsakoff patients; they have difficulties with attention and perception that may impair their performance on some remote memory tests.

(i) Senile Dementia: (*Senile* means old age) is characterised by deficits in many intellectual abilities - memory, attention, judgment and abstract thought, for example - that can occur in aged people. Personality changes - excessive dependence and irritability for instance - are common. Delusions - thoughts which have no basis in reality - and general disorientation - not knowing where one is in time or place - can also occur.

The amnesia in senile dementia is at first largely anterograde - the person has trouble remembering events that happened after the onset of the disease. Thus the old person with this disorder has trouble learning and cannot recall well what happened last month, yesterday or even a few hours ago. Memories of the years before the disease are largely intact until the brain damage becomes widespread and severe.

Senile dementia is usually the result of a reduction in blood flow to the brain. Most of the patients with this disorder have brain arteriosclerosis - narrowing of the small arteries of the brain due to fatty accumulation in them. Arteriosclerosis deprives brain cells of adequate supplies of oxygen and nutrients so that some cells die and others malfunction the brain is said to atrophy.

Normal ageing has its problems too, but the typical forgetfulness of old age is hardly severe enough to be called amnesia. In normal ageing, the memory problem, like that in senile dementia, centres largely on the storage of relatively recent events, it is anterograde in nature. But, in marked contrast to senile dementia patients, normal old people are able to compensate for their mild memory problems they try to do less and thus put a smaller burden on their information - processing systems they provide themselves with reminder cues, perhaps by writing down what is to be remembered and they organise their lives into routines so that fewer new things need to be remembered. In other words normal old people adopt adaptive memory strategies.

Primary degenerative dementia has many of the same characteristics as senile dementia. A major difference is that the symptoms often begin in middle age. Alzheimer's disease is a form of primary degenerative dementia in which there is a cluster of specific degenerative brain changes of unknown origin. Some evidence indicates that the Alzheimer's disease is related to deficiencies in the brain neurotransmitter chemical acetylcholine.

The tragedy of Alzheimer's disease is that it begins relatively early in life and unlike senile dementia, where death quickly ends the suffering life continues with progressive mental deterioration. The amnesia, for instance, often goes from a relatively mild anterograde memory problem to a profound anterograde and retrograde deficit - both the recent and remote past are largely gone.

Psychologists and other scientists, in near future may unravel the biochemical code of memory with new and sophisticated research techniques for the benefit of persons suffering from various kinds of memory disorders.

9

Mental Hygiene and Memory

> A great memory does not make a mind, any more than a dictionary is a piece of literature.
>
> —*John Henry Newman*

> Bad memory has its root in bad attention.
>
> —*Old Proverb*

According to Herman Ebbinghaus set out to study memory as simple cognitive function, uncomplicated by the meanings of the material to be remembered, or the expectations or characteristics of the person remembering. He used lists of 'nonsense syllables' which were pronounceable lists of letters; specifically, consonant-vowel-consonant trigrams, such as MAB, LOD. The idea was that these items, being meaningless could not be associated with each other, or with anything the person already knew. Research revealed some basic properties of memory. One of these is the 'serial position effect'. When a list of items is presented for learning, we are more likely to recall items early in the list (primacy effect) and items at the end of the list (recency effect) than items in the middle of the list. Bartlett used material rich in meaning, typically, stories and examined the nature of omissions and errors made when people retold the story. For Bartlett, active memory was characterized by 'effort after meaning'. It is only in second half of the 20th century, memory came to be viewed within the general cognitive framework if 'information processing' which combined aspects of two earlier approaches. Cognition was linkened to the operations of a computer that receives, manipulates, stores, and outputs information. At the same time it allows for previous knowledge and other sensory inputs to affect what is in the memory in various ways. William James stated that one's native retentiveness is unchangeable. Memory does not grow by exercise, as his experiments indicated, but it can be improved by improving one's methods of observation and learning. He proposed a primary memory that stores transient memories, and a secondary memory that stores information over long periods. An elaborate extension of this was the 'modal model' proposed in the 1960s by Atkinson and Shiffrin. Information is briefly saved in 'raw' form in an appropriate 'sensory register'. Research showed that much more information is available from the sensory register immediately after stimulus presentation than is available a few seconds later.

Fundamental Aspects

It is to be remembered that without memory there would be no learning. We would react to each occurrence of a situation as though it had not yet been experienced, each performance would require relearning. At the same time, without learning there would be nothing to remember. We might say that learning is the process of 'building up' memories for future use. While memory concerns the storage and retrieval of this information in the context of the following discussion, learning has been referred to as trace formation, memory as trace storage, and transfer of training as trace utilization.

Tracing the memory

Awareness of anything cannot be retained unless relevant earlier experience had produced some kind of change in the nervous system, a change often referred to as 'memory trace' or 'neurogram' or an 'engram' - to represent the neural basis of retention. Although this construct involves no specific assumptions about what structures of functions are modified it is believed that the engram may involve modifications analogous to the molecular changes which take place in a magnet recording tape.

'Memory' involves the making of an impress record of this impression and the re-entry of this record into consciousness as recall and recognition. . . . The human brain is composed of some 10 billion nerve cells, more or less alike, which interact in various ways. Each cell contributes to behavior and presumably to mental activity by firing impulses or failing to fire. All the phenomena of memory must be explained in terms of the temporal and spatial patterns of these discharges.

If experience is to modify behavior, the activity of neurons connected with an experience must be such as to alter their subsequent activity patterns. Two general questions must be asked regarding memory trace:

1. Does memory depend on a continuing activity or some static residue, some structural alteration, left behind by past activity ?
2. Is the structural trace (or dynamic process) for each memory located in a particular region of the brain or are memory traces subdued through the brain in some way ?

The answer to the first question suggests that memory is the static residue of past activity in a neural pathway. Thus each learning trial involves reactivating the same neural circuit. Eventually the circuit is in some sense permanently modified and therefore, when it is stimulated only partially later, the entire circuit is activated.

Memory as the process by which we encode, store and retrieve information.

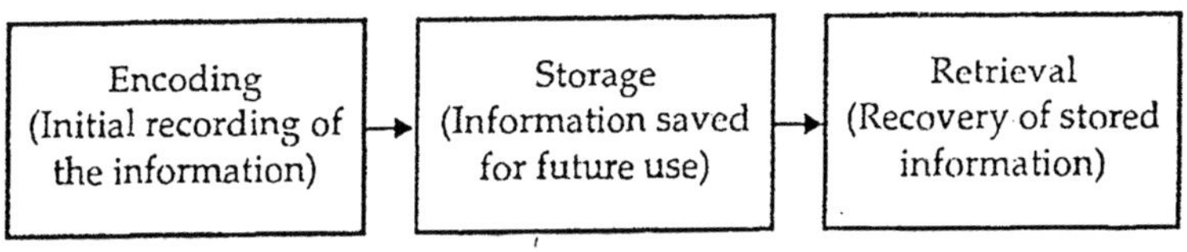
Encoding
(Initial recording of the information)
Storage
(Information saved for future use)
Retrieval
(Recovery of stored information)

Each of the three parts of this definition - encoding, storage and retrieval - represents a different process, which you can think of as analogous to a computers keyboard (encoding) disk (storage) and screen (retrieval). And only if all three processes have operated will you experience success and be able to recall the body of water on which Bombay is located: Arabian Sea.

Forgetting is essential to the proper functioning of memory. The ability to forget inconsequential details about experiences, people, and objects allows us to avoid being burdened and distracted by trivial stores of meaningless data. Furthermore, forgetting permits us to combine similar recollections and forms general impressions and recollections. For example, it would not be useful to form separate memories of the way friends look every time we saw them. Consequently we tend to forget their clothing, facial blemishes, and other unimportant that change from one occasion to the next. Instead our memories are based on a summarization of various important features, a far more economical use of our memory capabilities.

Systems of Memory

Psychologists divide memory into three types: Sensory; Short-term and Long-term memory.

(a) *Sensory memory* is the momentary lingering of sensory information after a stimulus has been removed. If you touch the palm of your hand with the point of a pencil, for example, you continue to feel the sensation for several seconds after the point is withdrawn. That momentary storage of tactile information is just one example of sensory storage systems for each of our different senses. We can store a great deal of information in these sensory registers, but only for an instant or so.

(b) *Short-term memory* is far more durable than sensory memory. Short- term memory contain the contents of your conscious awareness: what you are actively thinking about at any particular time. If your are trying to retain a phone number you have just looked up, if a tune keeps playing itself in your mind, if you recall the image of someone you know, you are processing this information through short term memory. Short term memory, is not just a passive storehouse of data, as older conceptions of it some times implied. Rather, it is a dynamic arena for processing information - for thinking, reasoning and solving problems. That is why today many cognitive psychologists prefer to call it active memory or working memory. Working memory system holds only a limited amount of information at any one time and its contents fade in about twenty seconds if they are not actively renewed.

(c) *Long term memory,* in contrast, can store things definitely without active effort. It can be thought of as a library of information and its capacity is believed to be limitless.

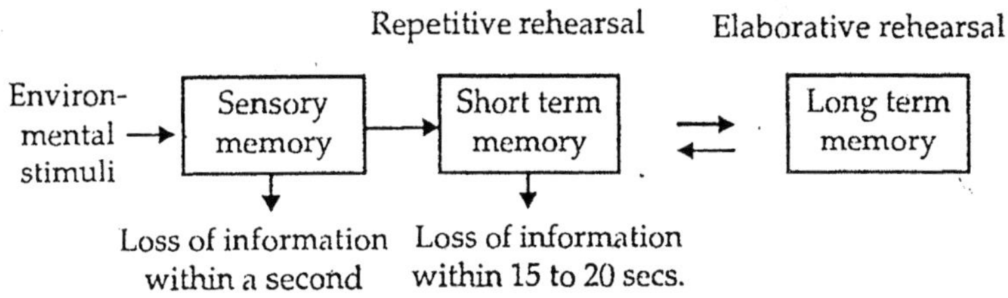

Sensory memory

Have a look for just an instant at the pattern of letters and numbers in the figure then close your eyes and try to list out loud as many as you can. You will probably find that your powers to recall are rather disappointing. In fact, the results of many carefully controlled experiments show that most people can remember only about four or five of twelve unrelated items that are flashed to them very briefly. Yet such findings seem to contradict everyday experience. When we glance quickly at something and then look away, we are usually left with the impression of a complete and accurate image, however fleeting that image may be.

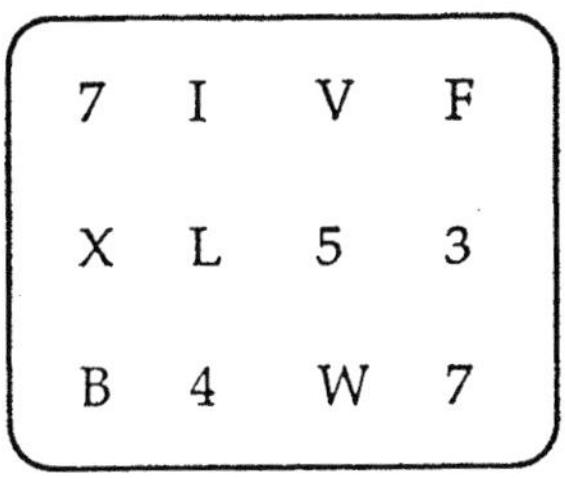

George Sperling (1960) conducted a series of clever and now classic studies on sensory memory. Sperling, briefly exposed people to a series of 12 letters arranged in the following patterns. When exposed to this array for just 1/20th second most people could accurately recall only 4 or 5 of the letters.

F	T	Y	C
K	D	N	L
Y	W	B	M

Although they knew they had seen more, the memory of rest of the letters had faded by the time they reported the first few letters. It was passive, then that the information had initially been accurately stored in sensory memory, but during the time it took to verbalize the first four or five letters the memory of the other letters faded. To test that possibility, Sperling conducted an experiment in which a high, medium or low tone sounded just after a person had been exposed to the full pattern of letters. People were told to report the letters in the highest line if a high tone were sounded, the middle line, if the medium tone occurred, or the lowest line at the sound of the low tone. Because the tone occurred after the exposure, people had to rely on their memory to report the correct row. The results of the study clearly showed that people had been storing the complete pattern in memory. They were accurate in their recollection of the letters in the line that had been indicated by the tone, regardless of whether it was the top, middle or bottom line.

Obviously all the lines that had seen had been stored in sensory memory. By gradually lengthening the time between the presentation of visual pattern and the tone, Serling was able to determine with some accuracy the length of time that information was stored in sensory memory. The ability to recall a particular row of pattern when a tone was sounded declined progressively as the period between visual exposure and tone increased. This decline continued until the period reached about one second in duration, at which point the row could not be recalled accurately at all. Sperling concluded that the entire visual image was stored in sensory memory for less than a second. In such, sensory memory operates as a kind of snapshot that stores information which may be of a visual, auditory or other sensory nature - for a brief moment of time. But it is as if each snapshot, immediately after being taken, is destroyed and replaced with a new one.

Short-term memory

Our working memory- because the information that is stored briefly in our sensory memory consists of representations of raw sensory stimuli it is not meaningful to us. In order for us to make sense of it and to allow for the possibility of long term retention, the information must be transferred to the next stage of short term memory. Shrot term memory is the memory store in which material first has meaning although the maximum length of retention is relatively short.

The specific process by which sensory memories are transformed into short term memories is not yet clear. Specific amount of information that can be held in short term memory has been identified: 7 items or chunks of information, with variations up to + or - to chunks. A chunk is a meaningful grouping of stimuli that can be stored as a unit in short term memory.

According to George Miller (1956) it could be individual letters, as in the following list :

C N Q M W N T

Each letter here qualifies as a separate chunk, and as there are seven of them they are easily held in short term memory.

But a chunk might also consist of larger categories, such as words or other meaningful units. For example, consider the following list of 21 letters:

T W A C I A A B C C S S M T V U S A N B C

Clearly, because the list exceeds seven chunks, it is difficult to recall the letters after one exposure. But suppose they were presented to you as follows:

TWA CIA ABC CBS MTV USA NBC

In this case, even though there are still 21 letters, it would be possible to store them in memory, since they represent only seven chunks.

The reason the task suddenly became so simple was that shapes could be grouped together into one chunk - a word that we all recognize, rather than being separate symbols with no meaning, they are recorded as just one chunk. Chunks can vary in size from single letters or numbers to categories that are far more complicated, the specific number of what constitutes a chunk varies according to one's past experience. Although it is possible to remember seven or so relatively complicated sets of information entering short term memory, the information cannot be held there very long. Just how short term is short term memory? Anyone who has looked up a telephone number at a pay phone, struggled to find coins and forgotten the number at the sound of the dial tone knows that information in short term memory does not remain there terribly long.

Rehearsal: is the repetition of information that has entered short term memory. Rehearsal accomplishes two things. First, as long as the information is repeated it is kept alive in short term memory. More important, however, rehearsal allows is to transfer the material into long term memory. Whether the transfer is made from short - to - long term memory seems to depend largely on the kind of rehearsal that is carried out.

If the material is simply repeated over and over again - as we might do with a telephone number while we rush from the telephone booth to the telephone - it is kept current in short term memory, but it will not necessarily be placed in long term memory. Instead as soon as we stop dialing, the number is likely to be replaced by other information and will be completely forgotten. On the other hand, if the information in short term memory is rehearsed using a process called elaborative rehearsal, it is much more likely to be transferred into long term memory. Elaborative rehearsal occurs when the material is considered and organized in some fashion.

The organization might include expanding the information to make it fit into a logical framework, linking it to another memory, turning it into an image and transforming it in some other way. For example a list of vegetables to be purchased at a store could be woven together in memory as items being used to prepare an elaborate salad. By organizational strategies called mnemonics, we can vastly improve our retention of information.

Working memory : the components of short term memory:

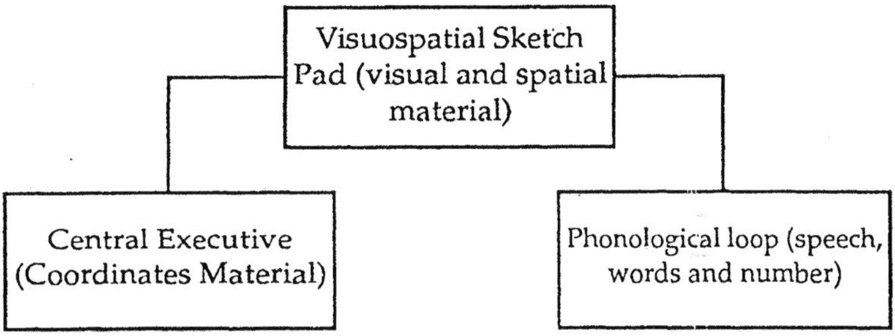

Though short term memory has traditionally been considered as a single system, more recent evidence suggests that it may actually consist of several components. According to Alan Baddeley (1992-93) Short term memory is better thought of as a three part working memory as shown in the figure above. In this view, one component is the central executive which coordinates the material to focus on during reasoning and decision making. The central executive makes use of two sub-components. The visuospatial scratch pad and the phonological loop. The visuospatial scratch pad concentrates on visual and spatial information while the phonological loop is responsible for holding and manipulating material relating to speech, words and numbers.

Long-term memory

Material that makes its way from short term memory to long term memory enters a store house of almost unlimited capacity. Like a new book delivered to a library, the information in LTM is filed and catalogued so that it can be retrieved when we need it.

Evidence of the existence of long term memory as distinct from short term memory, comes from a number of sources. For example people with certain kinds of brain damage have no lasting recall of new information following the damage, although people and events stored in memory prior to the injury remain intact. Because short term memory following the injury appears to be operative - new material can be recalled for a very brief period and because information enclosed and stored prior to the injury is recalled, we can infer that there are two distinct types of memory one for short term memory and one for long term memory.

The modules of memory

Although long term memory initially was viewed as a unitary entity, most research now suggests that it is composed of several different components or memory modules. Each of these modules is related to a separate memory system in the brain.

1. *Declarative memory:* is for factual information ; names, facts, dates and the like
2. *Procedural memory:* (Nondeclarative memory) refers to memory for skills and habits such as riding a bike or hitting a baseball.

Information about things is stored in declarative memory. Information regarding how to do things is stored in procedural memory.

Declarative memory can be further subdivided into semantic and episodic.

Semantic memory is memory for general knowledge and facts about the world, as well as memory for the rules of logic for deducing other facts. Because of semantic memory, we remember that 2 x 2 = 4, the spelling of words and codes of places etc.

Episodic memory is memory for the biographical details of our individual lives. Our memories of what we have done and the kinds of experiences we have had constitute episodic memory.

Long Term Memory
- Declarative factual
  - Semantic general
  - Episodic personal
- Procedural skills and habits

Episodic memories can be surprisingly detailed. It can provide information from events that happened long in the past.

Semantic memory consists of association between mental representation of various pieces of information.

Related information helps priming us to recall information that we are otherwise unable to recollect. In priming, prior presentation of information subsequently makes it easier to recall related items, even when we have no conscious memory of original information.

The discovery that people have memories about which they are unaware has been an important one. It has led to speculation that two forms of memory, explicit and implicit may exist side by side. Explicit memory refers to intentional or conscious recollection of information. When we try to remember a name or date we are using explicit memory. Implicit memory refers to memories of which people are not consciously aware, but which can affect subsequent performance and behavior.

Retrieval from Long term memory

Most people can read at a steady rate of 300 to 600 words per minute, or 5 to 10 words per second. This skill requires an amazingly efficient system for retrieving the meaning of words. But because we are so accustomed to our remarkable powers of information retrieval, we seldom stop to think how truly impressive they are. Psychologists have studied two kinds of retrieval from long-term storage: *Recognition* and *Recall.* Recognition involves deciding whether you have ever encountered a particular stimulus before. Identifying a suspect in a police line-up is an example of recognition. Recall in contrast, entails retrieving specific pieces of information usually guided by retrieval cues.

We have all had the frustrating experience of being unable to recall something that we know is stored in memory. Some times this experience produces what is called the tip-of-the-tongue phenomenon. We feel that an answer is poised to emerge, but some how we just cannot get it out. How do we try these uncomparitive facts? We use a variety of retrieval cues based on bits of information about the target word that we are able to recall. When shown a picture of popular actor and asked to remember the name of one of his films, we seem to create a number of retrieval path ways to it. These pathways typically involve both sounds and associated facts and meanings. Since recall always involves a search through memory to find the correct response, is recall necessarily more difficult than recognition? Frequently it is. Most students find that multiple choice question (recognition tests) are substantially easier than fill-in-the-blanks (recall tests). The reason is that in multiple choice test the answer is right there before you. All you have to do is match it with information learned previously. So as long as you are familiar with the correct answer the possibilities offered are not confusingly similar, you will probably make the right choice.

Use of Mnemonics devices: (Greek word - meaning memory) Some simple techniques can greatly improve almost anyone's powers of recall.

1. Shopping lists
2. First-letter memory aids
3. Diary
4. Rhymes
5. Place method

6. Writing on your hand
7. The story method
8. Mentally retracing a sequence of events
9. Alarm clock
10. Kitchen timer with alarm
11. Memos
12. Face-name association
13. Calendars, wall charts, year planners, display boards
14. Asking other people to remember things for you
15. Leaving objects in special or unusual places so that they act as reminders

Organizations: How much a person can retrieve from his data storage system appears to be largely the result of his organization of the material. This observation suggests the importance of shaping a large mass of information into some sort of meaningful structure if one is to be able to recall most of it. This procedure is especially helpful in answering college examination questions in which there are often few specific cues to aid the student in retrieving information. The student in order to remember may, for example, take the first letter of the words and coin an anagram (VIBGYOR, UNESCO, UNICEF).

Associations: William James once said that the secret of a good memory is *'forming diverse and multiple associations with every fact we care to retain. But this forming of associations with a fact, what is it, but thinking about the fact as much as possible ? Briefly, then of two men with the same outward experiences and the same amount of mere native tenacity, the one who 'thinks' over his experiences most, and wears them into systematic relations with each other, will be the one with best memory.* The encoding process is highly subjective and unique.

To decrease forgetting, one should associate newly acquired information with some cue which will be readily available for example the spelling for George could be remembered as 'Ge' or 'ge'.

Tips to Remember

If you want to remember what you need to know in courses or in your work, practice the following:

1. You should spend a great deal of your time (study) in Elaborative rehearsal: Ask yourself what you have just read, what the new concepts and terms are, and how they relate to other things you know or are learning. Studies show that it is effective to spend atleast half of your study time in such rehearsal.
2. Plan a study schedule that you can stick to. During the time you set aside for study, work at it instead of talking to friends or watching TV out of the corner of your eye. If you study hard during your scheduled times, you will find that you have plenty of time for your friends and amusement.
3. Review before the examination. You will have forgotten many of the details you learned. Relearn the way you learned them in the first place and key your review for the type of examination. If the examination will be stressing recall, as in an essay examination, spend a good deal of your time rehearsing major ideas and the experiments that support them. Trying to think of what the questions will be ahead of time and practicing your answers to them is a good idea. If the examination is to be multiple-choice, or some other objective type, be sure you have mastered the definitions of the terms and can recognise the correct definition when you see them.
4. Try to get some idea of how well you remember the material. In other words, get some feedback. If you study by breaking the material into parts, try to get some feedback after you study each part. Go back over what you have studied and using the headings as retrieval cues, ask yourself what is under each heading. Turn to the terms at the end of the chapter

and ask yourself for definitions of the appropriate terms. Feedback will tell you both what you have mastered and where you are weak when you have finished a chapter test yourself on it and do some additional work on any weak spots. By testing yourself, you will also be practicing your retrieval skills.

5. As you rehearse elaboratively, you will also be providing yourself with retrieval cues, you will be giving your own subjective organisation that will be important when you try to recall what you are learning, if you can, form visual images of abstract ideas.

10

Infants' Movements

From the beginning of independent life, movement is the infant's natural response to all influences. And, more than this, Bain and Preyer seem to have made out their case, that from the outset there are movements which are spontaneous, due to discharge of the motor centres unsolicited by definite external stimulations. At any rate, no observation made after birth can decide the question one way or the other whether sensation or movement is the earlier fact in ontogenetic development. It remains for the embryologists to continue their work, and this is where Preyer's results get their principal value.

Reflexes. — In regard to movements more properly reflex and responsive, we may record a few detached observations on my child. Carefully planned experiments with her, made in the ninth month, showed the native walking reflex — alternative movement of the legs — very strongly marked. We held her by the body, having made the legs quite free, in a position which allowed the bare feet to rest lightly upon a smooth table. The reflex seemed to come somewhat suddenly, for ~ to the middle of the eighth month we could not discover more than a single alternation; and this I had determined not to take as evidence, since it might well arise by chance. But, in the ninth month, I observed as many as three and four well-regulated alternations, in succession. At first most of these movements were the reverse of the natural walking movements, being oftenest such as would carry the child backward. This, however, passed away. I have the following note on June 13, 1890, the child being one day short of nine months old: " Walking movements, 3 to 4 alternations, backwards oftenest, but tending rapidly to forward movements; later, 2 experiments, each showing 3 to 4 alternations forwards very plainly;" and on June 19: "Fine activity in walking reflex — good alternations, but more backwards than forwards — clearly reflex, from stimulus to the soles." It is easy to see that this backward alternation might be due to some accident of stimulation or discharge when the reflex was first called out; a tendency which early efforts at creeping would soon correct. Yet in H.'s case, it was so marked that for a period she preferred to creep backward.

A few observations were made also upon unilateral reflexes. A gentle touch with finger or feather on the cheek, or beside the nose, or upon the ear, when H. was sleeping quietly upon her back, called out always the hand on the same side. After two or three such irritations, her sleep became troubled and she turned upon the bed, or used both hands to rub the place stimulated. Tickling of the sole of the foot also, besides causing a reaction in the same foot, tended to bring about a movement of the hand on the same side. These observations, not a large number, were made in the sixth, seventh, and eighth months.

In order to test the growth of voluntary control over the muscles of the hand and fingers, I determined to observe the phenomena of H.'s attempts at drawing and writing, for which she showed great fondness as soon as imitation was well fixed. Selecting a few objects well differentiated in outline, — animals which she had already learned to recognize and name after a fashion, — we drew them one by one on paper and let her imitate the 'copy.' The results I have in a series of 'drawings' of hers, extending from the last week of her nineteenth month to the middle of the twenty seventh month. The results show that, with this child, up to the beginning of the twenty-seventh month there was no connection apparent between a mental picture in consciousness and the movements made by the hands and fingers in attempting to draw it. The 'drawing' was simply the vaguest and most general imitation of the teacher's movements, not the tracing of a mental picture. And the attempt was no better when a 'copy' was made by myself on the paper — a rough outline drawing of a man, etc. There was no semblance of conformity between the child's drawing and the copy. Further, while she could identify the copy and name the animal, she could not identify her own effort, except so far as she remembered what object she set out to make.

With it all there was on her face an expression of dissatisfaction with her later attempts, similar to that which one observes in the efforts of the year-old to speak. My little girl would hide her head after making a drawing, extend the pencil to me, and say, 'Papa make man.' It seemed to indicate a sense of what was expected beyond the ability to attain the process of accomplishing it.

In the nature of the movements which the child made in this series of drawings, there is marked change and development which may be briefly described. There is growth from angular straight lines to curves, from movements one way exclusively to reverse movements, and an increasing tendency to complex intricate figures, which last probably results from greatly increased ease, variety, and rapidity of movement. At first she made only sweeping 'arm movements,' then began to flex the wrist somewhat, and toward the end of the series given above, as is evident in the figures, with no teaching, manipulated the pencil with her fingers considerably. This seems to give support to the opinion of professional writing teachers that the 'arm movement' is most natural and effective for purposes of penmanship.

Further, all her curves were made by movements from

left to right going upward and from right to left downward, like the movements of the hands of a clock. This is the method of our usual writing as contrasted with 'back-hand.' She also preferred lateral to vertical movements on the paper. Her most frequent and easy 'drawing' consisted of a series of rapid right and left strokes almost parallel to one another, constituting very narrow and long loops.

But early in the twenty-seventh month a change came. We drew a rough human figure, naming the parts in succession as they were made: she suddenly seemed to catch the idea of tracing each part, and she now for the first time began to make figures with vertical and horizontal proportion; i.e. she followed the order she saw me take: 'head' (circle), 'body' (ellipse) below, 'legs' (two straight lines) further below, 'hands' (two lines) at the sides of the body. It was all done in the crudest fashion, as would be expected from the lack of muscular co-ordination. But the fact was unmistakable that with the simplification of the figure by breaking it up into parts had come also the idea of tracery imitation, and its imperfect execution. By the 'idea' of tracery imitation, we mean the sense of connection between what was visually in her own consciousness and the movement of her own hand or pencil. The visual pictures or copies had been there in all her previous trials, and so had the hand movements, both the sight of them and the muscular sensations; but there had been no sense of a connection between them and agreement in the result when they were compared.

As yet, however, it was limited to two or three copies — objects which she saw me make. That it was now not simply imitation of my movements is evident from the fact that she did not imitate my movements: she looked intently upon the figure which we made, not at my movements, and then strove to imitate the figure with movements of her own very different from mine. But she had not generalized the idea away from particular figures, for she could not trace at all an altogether new figure in right lines. Further, she traced these particular figures just as well without written copies before her: here, therefore, is the rise of the tracery imitation of the child's own mental picture — a fact of great theoretical interest.

A curious phenomenon, which has been noticed also by Passy in the drawings of much older children, was evident in H.'s attempts to extend her drawings to other objects. This is the tendency to neglect the new object or copy and substitute for it in whole or part some drawing which she had already learned to make. For example, having analyzed man after me into head, body, legs, and arms, this became her scheme for drawing all other creatures. When told to draw a bird after a copy set before her, she gave it all these features, conforming them in a measure to the general shape of a bird, but putting two strokes at the sides for *arms.* We shall say more about this fact in the next section in discussing the origin of handwriting; it is also suggestive in connection with the rise of the general notion.

Interpretation of Tracery Imitation: the Origin of Handwriting

It is easily seen that the fact to which we have given the name 'tracery imitation' lies at the basis of handwriting. It is clear that handwriting is acquired by imitation of a copy. Each letter is acquired by the tracing out of a form put before the child. There are two very distinct steps, however, in the acquisition of handwriting, the first of which is tracery imitation of an external copy; and the second is the similar imitation of a memory picture or form. The relation of these two things to each other and, with that, the general theory of handwriting, requires farther analysis. We shall depict in some detail the progress of this function, since it serves to illustrate the general theory of the development of muscular control worked out in a later chapter.

The preliminary question as to how the child gets its visual apprehension of form may be answered, and has been, in two ways. Some hold that the actual form or arrangement of the retinal elements stimulated by the rays of light from the object seen is conveyed to consciousness by a series of 'local signs' — distinct quality of some kind which serves to distinguish each visual or anatomical point from every other. Others hold that the eye explores~in its movement the outline of the object, and a constant succession of sensations of eye movement thus represents the particular form explored. It is safe to say that, whether one or both of these causes operate to give the child its form intuition, we can still say that there is a constant series of sensations from the eyes, which can be run over in one direction, or the reverse; this we may call the 'visual form series,' v, v', v'', in the analysis of handwriting.

But the child, in setting out to draw, moves his- hand, thus getting sensations from the hand itself according to its locality at this moment and at that. If you consider the hand as moving slowly, it will be evident that there are touch sensations, joint sensations, muscle-tension sensations, etc., giving together a certain massive sense of the locality of the hand as it goes from place to place. With no care as to the exact character of these sensations, we may yet say that there is a series which is constant for the drawing of the outline of a plane figure; this series we may call the 'muscular form series,' denoted by m, m', m''.

But, further, the child has other means of finding out about movements than by the sensations from his own hand and arm. He sees other people's movements and his own. In this case of drawing, he is instructed in holding his pencil, sees his teacher move his pencil over the paper, sees his own arm and hand and pencil-point in each case. This, it is evident, gives a more or less exact additional series of eye sensations, according as the child is able by frequent following of the movements of others and himself to appropriate each such set of movements to a regular visual form. This third series of sensations, in a particular case, we may call the 'optical movement series, *o*, *o*′, *o*″, etc.

It is evident that the acquisition of writing involves all of these three series; and it is easy to show that they are all present in our most rapid and careless writing. If one shut his eyes and write, he preserves the general form of the letters, but they are badly made compared with those which he makes when he sees his pen and follows its movement. This shows his dependence upon the o series. But he can still very greatly improve his penmanship if his paper be ruled, or more again if he write after a well-written copy; this shows the dependence, relatively slight, upon the *v* series. As to the revival of the *v* series also, as copies to which to conform, cases of verbal blindness show that lesions of the optical brain centre may make it impossible for one to write at all. Further, if we try to write with the skin benumbed with cold, or on a surface which yields, the letters are made without form and thrown out of their due proportion. This in turn shows the continual presence of the m series.

That a child gets his visual form (*v*) series first is proved from his recognition and even naming of figures, pictures, etc., before he draws them or sees them drawn. These series are at first few, but he gradually adds to them as the range of his exploration becomes wider and as familiar objects become in his experience more and more familiar. There is a constant tendency, therefore, from the random wandering of the eyes over many forms and over shapeless things, to concentration on interesting, familiar, and regular forms of things. So we may say there is a continual growth and upbuilding of different *v* series.

This is at the expense of the optical movement (*o*) series, as may be seen from the following considerations: At first the child follows all movements, that he sees, of himself and of others, with equal attention — his eye is a slave to movement anywhere and everywhere — his attention is reflex and visual. He looks closely at his own movements.

Now there, in this association, is the rise of 'tracery imitation' in its crudest form; this reversal of association between the *o* and the *v* elements. Its characteristics, as imitation, are merely the vaguest indications of direction and proportion. It utilizes no constant m series; that is, no constant detailed series of hand and arm movements, but only the up and down, and right and left, movements acquired by the child in its early random exercises, together with whatever more definite movements education may have produced. To interpret it, H.'s ability suddenly to 'imitate' my drawing of a man was largely the discovery that by a series of ordinary movements of her own which she saw (*o* element), and which her random practice had made easy, she could bring about, in a measure, what I did. Instead of her eye following the tracing left by the point of the pen (*v* series subordinated to *o* series), as formerly it did, she now found that her hand and pen, as she watched them, could follow the outline we had made, or her memory of it (*o* series subordinated to the *v* series).

Such as it is, however, tracery imitation is a long way from handwriting. And the essential difference is the introduction of sensations of movement (*m* series), whereby the operations of the hand are held in control. How, then, does the *m* series get its influence ?

Eye movements start in a chaotic random state, as we have seen, and only gradually take on the definite character of separate series, as the customary explorations, fixations, visual curiosities of experience serve to fix them. But arm movements are just the reverse. At first the arm is capable of very few movements, the elbow of one, and the fingers of none. Moreover, the joints are stiff, the movements to a degree inconvenient, and all ventures away from certain reactions provided for by native arrangements are painful and unsuccessful. This means that the child starts with certain very definite arm movements (*m* series). But this does not last. He gets limbered up. His *m* series gets broken into ur.its and recombined into new series. This is seen in the progress shown in H.'s series of drawings given above.

This prepares the way for a second victory of the *v* series. At first the hand must move in certain directions represented in consciousness by the series *m*, *m'*, *m"*, etc.; the eye can move in any direction indifferently; so the eye follows the hand.

Now certain muscular sensations (*m* elements) represent movements which, being also seen, have *o* elements attached to them. And we have already seen that tracery imitation requires a certain correspondence between relatively fixed *v* series and relatively free *o* series. The breaking up of the *m* series just described now makes it possible for more of these correspondences to occur, i.e. for more movements seen to describe figures seen. Now it is by the gradual increase of these correspondences, this practice and emphasis into habit, that handwriting is built up with much effort.

There is, therefore, an extremely close association between a visual figure series and the series of hand movements required to reproduce it. And this association between them is secured by the reproduction concomitantly through the seen hand movements (o series) of a real figure which conforms to the original visual ideal by which the whole is prompted.

It is easy to see, therefore, that in handwriting the movements made are controlled by two different but concurring agencies: first, the sensations in the arm and hand must be, point by point, those called for by the fast associations of movement with letter outlines. This tendency is actually so strong in the young child who has learned to make a few figures successfully, that it draws new objects like the old shapes, even when they are really very different, and in spite of close attention to the plain copies put before them. And, second, the figure which the eye takes in as the pen point inscribes it, must also agree, point by point, with the outline figure which is held in consciousness and aimed at.

With the further development of handwriting, the performance tends to become independent of sight. In swift writing we use our eyes mainly to keep on the line and on the paper, not to see that the letters are made properly. As far as we do examine them, it is only to see that they fall within the limits of legibility; and we know so well about what our hand can do, that we rarely have occasion to revise a word once written. The muscular series (*m* series) becomes so delicately adjusted to the needs of the memory image of figure, of letter, and of word (*v* series), that a further optical test (*o* series) is not required.

It is interesting to note, also, that this growing independence in the sensations of movement under practice and habit may go so far that the visual copy (*v* series) may be dispensed with altogether; this is shown to be true in pathological cases of alexia, or inability to read, which do not involve agraphia, or inability to write. In these cases we have the extreme motor type of verbal memory, emphasized by Stricker: persons who remember written words by the memory of the sensations involved in writing them.

A further fundamental question arises, however, when we come to examine the actual parallelism of the associated series of elements involved. How does it come about that the child is able to secure the agreement, term by term, between the elements of the v and the m series respectively — the agreement by which this association is established? How does he get v with m, v' with m', v'' with m'', in this regular way, and both in proper association with *o, o′, o″*, etc. ? This is the question of the possibility of any adaptation of movements to ends, whether voluntary or not. Its discussion is taken up later, and in that connection the general principles are given by which this case may be solved with others.

The kinds and varieties of agraphia — inability to write, from nervous lesion — are well classified, on the basis of impairment of one or more of the elements involved, by Goldscheider, in the paper already quoted. His explanation of mirror-writing is, however, so clearly a proof of the adequacy of the point in which his theory and mine agree, that we may briefly explain it.

Mirror-writing is the form of inscription which arises from tracing words with the left hand by an exact reduplication of the movements of the right hand, in a symmetrical way from the central point in front of the body, out toward the left. It produces a form of reversed writing which cannot be read until it is seen in a mirror. Many left-handed children tend to write in this way. Some adults, on taking a pen to write with the left hand, find they can write only in this way. Even those, like myself, to whom the movements seem, when thought of in visual terms, quite confusing and impossible, yet find, when they try to write with both hands together, in the air, from a central point right and left, that the left-hand mirror-writing movements are very natural and easy. Now, why is it?

If a man is of the so-called 'visual' type, i.e. if he depends mainly on his v series, recalling, in his writing, the look of the letters, etc., and by comparing it with the resulting writing, conforming his movement series to it, then any movements which violate the figure presented by visual memory are unintelligible. Such a man must reproduce, with his left hand, the visual images as produced by the right. That is, he must write from left to right with both hands, using visually symmetrical images. This represents the power of the *v* series to bring the movements of both hands into conformity to it. If, on the contrary, his *m* series has grown independent by practice, and he remembers written words not by the way they look mainly, but by the way it feels to write them — if he is of the so-called 'motor' type in his handwriting — then his left-hand writing must reproduce the series of muscular sensations, as his right-hand writing has established them. This represents the power of movements established by one hand to carry the other hand also with it in a symmetrical way. His left-hand position must duplicate at each moment his right-hand position, when he comes to try the experiment of writing in the air with both hands. This gives symmetrical movements with the two hands, which means mirror-writing with the left hand.

The following notice and criticism of Goldscheider's paper, may serve to show the difference between my theory and his, and at the same time sum up the foregoing discussion.

Goldscheider gives first a theoretical account of the origin of what is called 'tracery imitation' under the equivalent phrase *malende Reproduction*, endeavouring to account for the association between visual pictures (letters, figures, etc.) and the hand movements necessary to reproduce them (as in drawing, writing, etc.). He finds three factors or 'moments' in the rise of tracery imitation: *A*, an optical picture of the hand movements required for making the required figure (*optische Vorstellung der Handbewegung;* my *o* series), derived from the child's earlier sight of his own and others' hand movements; *B*, a series of new motor discharges strengthened by practice, felt as C, a series of sensations of actual movement, by which the discharges are regulated and controlled (*motorisches Bewegungsbild;* my *m* series). Moment *A* is clearly seen in the fact often remarked, that in writing with the eyes closed we still follow the pen point in its inscription of an optical outline. Further, in moment *A* there are two factors:

11

Suggestions

The rise of hypnotism in late years has opened the way to an entirely new method of mental study. The doctrine of reflexes was before largely physiological, and only pathological cases could be cited in evidence of a mechanism in certain forms of consciousness as well as out of it; and even pathological cases of extreme sensitiveness to casual suggestion from the environment or from other men did not receive the interpretation which the phenomena of hypnotic suggestion are now making possible, i.e. that suggestion by idea, or through consciousness, must be recognized to be as fundamental a kind of motor stimulus as the direct excitation of a sense organ. Nervous reflexes may work directly through states of consciousness, or be stimulated by them; these states of consciousness may be integral portions of such reflexes; and, further, a large part of our mental life is made up of a mass of such ideo-motor 'suggestions,' which are normally in a state of subconscious inhibition.

Janet defines suggestion as " a motor reaction brought about by language or perception." This narrows the field to certain classes of stimulations, well defined in consciousness, and overlooks the more subtle suggestive influences emphasized by the Nancy school of theorizers. Schmidkunz makes it: "die Herbeirufung eines Ereigrusses durch die Erweckung seines psychischen Bildes." This again makes a mental picture of the suggested 'event' in consciousness necessary, and, besides, does not rule out ordinary complex associations. It neglects the requirement insisted upon by Janet, i.e. that the stimulus be from without, as from hearing words, seeing actions, objects, etc. Wundt says: "Suggestion ist Association mit gleichzeitiger Verengerung des Bewusstseins auf die durch die Association angeregten Vorstellungen." In this definition Wundt meets the objection urged against the definition of suggestion in terms of complex association, by holding down the association to a 'narrowed consciousness'; but he, again, neglects the outward nature of the stimulus, and does not give an adequate account of how this narrowing of consciousness upon one or two associated terms, usually a sensori-motor association, is brought about. Ziehen: "In der Beibringung der Vorstellung liegt das Wesen der Suggestion." Here we have the sufficient recognition of the artificial and external source of the stimulation, but yet we surely cannot say that all such stimulations succeed in getting suggestive force. A thousand things suggested to us are rejected, scorned, laughed at. This is so marked a fact in current theory, especially on the pathological side, that we have found it convenient to use a special phrase for consciousness when in the purely suggestible condition, i.e. 'reactive consciousness.' The phrase 'conscious reflex' is sometimes used, but is not good as applied to these suggestive reactions; for they are cortical in their brain seat, and are not as definite as ordinary reflexes.

Physiological Suggestion

By 'suggestion' is understood ordinarily ideal or ideo-motor suggestion, — the origination from without of a motor reaction, by producing in consciousness the state which is ordinarily antecedent to that reaction; but observation of an infant for the first month or six weeks of its life leads to the conviction that its life is mainly physiological. The vacancy of consciousness as regards anything not immediately given as sensation, principally pleasure and pain, precludes the possibility of *ideal* suggestion as such. The infant at this age has no ideas in the sense of distinct memory images. Its conscious states are largely affective. Accordingly, when the reactions which are purely reflex, and certain random impulsive movements, are excluded, we seem to exhaust the contents of its motor consciousness.

Yet even at this remarkably early stage H. was found to be in a degree receptive of suggestion, — suggestion conveyed by repeated stimulation under uniform conditions. In the first place, the suggestions of sleep began to tell upon her before the end of the first month. Her nurse put her to sleep by laying her face down and patting gently upon the end of her spine. This position itself soon became not only suggestive to the child of sleep, but sometimes necessary to sleep, even when she was laid across the nurse's lap in what seemed to be an uncomfortable position.

This case illustrates what we mean by physiological suggestion. It shows the law of physiological habit as it borders on the conscious. No doubt some such effect would be produced by pure habit apart from consciousness; but, consciousness being present, its nascent indefinite states may be supposed to have a quality of suggestiveness, which works to increase the fixedness of the habit. Yet the fact of such a colouring of consciousness in connection with the growth of physiological habit is important rather as a transition to more evident suggestion.

The same kind of phenomena appear also in adult life. Positions given to the limbs of a sleeper lead to movements ordinarily associated with these positions. The sleeper defends himself, withdraws himself from cold, etc. Children learn gradually the reactions upon conditions of position, lack of support, etc., of the body, necessary to keep from falling out of bed, which adults have so perfectly. All secondary automatic reactions may be classed here, the sensations coming from one reaction, as in walking, being suggestions to the next movement, unconsciously acted upon. The state of consciousness at any stage in the chain of movements, if present at all, must be similar to the baby's in the case above, — a mere internal glimmering, whose reproduction, however brought about, reinforces its appropriate reaction.

The most we can say of such physiological suggestion is, that the conscious state is always present, and that the ordinary reflexes may be subsequently abbreviated and modified.

Professor Ribot says as much as this. "When a physiological state has become a state of consciousness, through this very fact it has acquired a particular character.... It has became a new factor in the psychic life of the individual — a result that can serve as a starting-point to some new (either conscious or unconscious) work." And again: "Volition is a state of consciousness . . . it marks a series, i.e. the possibility of being recommenced, modified, prevented. Nothing similar exists in regard to automatic acts that are not accompanied by consciousness.... Each state of consciousness . . . in relation to the future development of the individual, is a factor of the first order." Schneider, also, writing from the phylogenetic point of view, says: "All purely physiological movements serve a single definite purpose, are always the same; psychological movements, an the contrary, have the peculiarity that they serve *different* purposes, follow upon quite different stimulations, and adapt themselves to circumstances by combination and modification.... Otherwise we would not have any consciousness, for there would be no uşe for it.... So in connection with every movement which is accompanied by a phenomenon of consciousness, we may hold, that this phenomenon of consciousness is really necessary (*wirklich nothig ist*) for the determination of the movement."

A more positive pronouncement on the presence of consciousness in all reactions to which the term 'suggestion' may be applied is that of Moll. He says: " *There is no suggestion without consciousness.* It makes no difference whether the suggestion is made through imitation or by a command.... we must insist in opposition to Mendel that there is consciousness of what is suggested, and that this is the main point in the matter. A suggestion without consciousness is to me inconceivable."

In hypnotic experimentation, the influence of such subconscious or physiological suggestions is now generally recognized under the general doctrine of hyperaesthesia of the senses. Ochorowicz calls the general phenomenon of suggestion *ideoplasty*, and when no clear idea is necessary to the effect, as in my 'physiological' suggestion, he speaks Of 'physical ideoplasty.' He says: "We have *ideoplasty* whenever the thought alone of any functional modification determines such functional modification . . . the thought of yawning itself produces yawning, etc."

A particular observation made upon my child E. during her second year may serve to make clear this first stage of suggestion. She learned to go to sleep sucking her bottle, the rubber of which was left in her mouth while she slept. Now, at any sound, touch, or other sudden stimulation, such as the flaring up of the light, she began with more or less vigour to suck the bottle, giving no other sign of awaking whatever, and really not awaking, but only passing from a deeper sleep, or less consciousness, to a lighter sleep, or more consciousness. Now, as we interpret it, the stimulus, arousing more brain process, heightened the sleep or dream consciousness, brought out the sensations in the lips about the rubber, and these sensations by *physiological suggestion* set up the sucking movements. These movements in turn had their habitual influence in sending the child off into deep sleep again. Then, later, it is probable that even the lip sensations were not necessary; but the increased dynamogeny of the increased sensory consciousness simply poured itself into the lip-movement channels, since they were associated last and always with the conditions of sleep.

Sensori-motor Suggestion

These cases of suggestion may again be best illustrated from the phenomena of infancy, before a close definition is attempted. And first we may note some instances of what may be called *general suggestions* of this sort.

I. General. — Various Sleep Suggestions. — From the first month on, there was a deepening of the hold upon the child H. of the early method of inducing sleep. The nurse, in the meantime, added two nursery rhymes. Thus position, pats, and rhyme sounds were the suggesting stimuli. Not until the third month, however, was there any difference noticed when the same suggestions came from other persons. We ourself learned, during the fourth month, to put her to sleep, and learned with great difficulty, though pursuing the nurse's method as nearly as possible. Here, therefore, was a sleep suggestion from the *personality* of the nurse, — her peculiar voice, touch, etc.,—of which mention is made more fully below. At this time we assumed exclusive charge of putting H. to sleep, in order to observe the phenomena more closely. For a month or six weeks we made regular improvement, reducing the time required from three-quarters of an hour to half an hour, finding it easier at night than at midday. This indicated that darkness had already become an additional sleep suggestion, probably because it shut out the whole class of sensations from sight, thus reducing the attention to stimulations which were monotonous.

In the following month (sixth), we reduced the time required, day or night, to about a quarter of an hour, on an average. In this way we found it possible to send her off to sleep at any hour of the night that she might wake and cry out.

We then determined to omit the patting, and endeavour to bring on sleep by singing only. The time was at first lengthened, then greatly shortened. We now found it possible (sixth to seventh month) to put her to sleep, when she waked in the dark, by a simple refrain repeated monotonously two or three times. In the meantime she was developing active attention, and resisted all endeavours of her nurse and mother, who had been separated from her through illness, very stubbornly for hours, while she would go to sleep for myself, even when most restless, in from fifteen to thirty minutes. This result required sometimes firm holding down of the infant and a determined expression of countenance.

At the end of the year, this treatment being regular, she would voluntarily throw herself in the old position at a single word from me, and go to sleep, if only patted uniformly, in from four to ten minutes. This continued through the second year; even when she was so restless that her nurse was unable to keep her from gaining her feet, and when she screamed if forced by her to lie down. The sight of myself was sufficient to make her quiet; and in five minutes, rarely more, she was sound asleep.

This illustrates, as conclusively as could be desired, the passage of purely physiological over into sensory suggestion; and this is all that we care, in this connection, to emphasize.

Food and Clothing Suggestion. — H. gave unmistakable signs of response to the sight of her food-bottle as early, at least, as the fourth month, probably a fortnight earlier. The reactions were a kind of general movement toward the bottle, especially with the hands, a brightening of the face, and crowing sounds. It is curious that the rubber on the bottle seemed to be the point of identification, the bottle being generally not responded to when the rubber was removed. This was also true of E., to whom the rubber alone without the bottle became a remarkable quieting agent, as we have already mentioned. The sight of the bottle, also, was suggestive much earlier than the touch of it with her hands.

H. began to show a vague sense of the use of her articles of clothing about the fifth month, responding at the proper time, when being clothed, by ducking her head, extending her hand or withdrawing it. About this time she also showed signs of joy at the appearance of her mittens, hood, and cloak, before going out.

II. Suggestions of Personality. — It was a poet, no doubt, who first informed us that the infant inherits a peculiar sensibility for its mother's face, —a readiness to answer it with a smile. This is all poetic fancy. It is true that the infant does smile very early; E. clearly smiled at me on her seventh day and at her mother on the ninth. But it is probably a purely reflex indication of agreeable organic sensation. When the child does begin to show partiality for mother or nurse, it is because the kind treatment it has already experienced in connection with the face has already brought out the same smile before in this organic way; the mother's face, that is, grows to suggest the smile. At first it is not the face alone, but the personality, *the presence*, to which the child responds; and of more special suggestion, the voice is first effectual, then touch, as in the case of sleep above, and then sight. Such suggestions are among the most important of infancy, serving as elements in the growth of the consciousness of self and of external reality, as we shall have occasion to see later on.

Delaying for the moment the further analysis of this remarkable class of suggestions, the question occurs, are not these so-called 'suggestions' simply cases of the association of ideas? We think we are warranted in answering, 'No'; for the reason that it is not an associated idea that is brought up; unless we are prepared to enlarge the ordinary conception of association to include phenomena of the vaguest psychological meaning. The muscular movement is produced without the production of an idea of that movement, largely through native pathways of discharge, or by the production of organic conditions, such as sleep, which involve muscular conditions. Can we say that the sleep suggestions first bring up an idea or image of the sleep condition, or that the bottle brings up an idea of the movements of grasping, or even of the sweet taste? We think the case is more direct. The energy of stimulation passes over into the motor reaction through the medium of the conscious state; although the conscious state is undoubtedly enveloped in an envelope or fringe of organic and muscular sensation which is of marked hedonic quality. Further, as will appear clearer below, it is not an association plus a suggestion, or an association plus an association, as current atomistic doctrines of association would lead us to expect. We cannot say that pleasure or pain always intervenes between the present state of consciousness and the motor reaction, i.e. mother's face, pleasure recalled, expression of pleasure, or present bottle, sweet taste, movements to reach. We believe all this is quite artificial and unnatural. The most that can be said is that the conscious state as a whole, with its hedonic colouring, serves to bring about a modification of the reaction, whether it be a native one, or one established by association or habit.

The phenomenon of 'personality-suggestion,' to which we may now return, is so important in the growth of the child's consciousness of himself, of his belief in realities about him, and of his social life, that it should be closely scrutinized. This is the more important because such an analysis has never been made upon the basis of actual observation of children. The treatment which follows is based upon most detailed and watchful inspection of H. and E., together with careful but less intimate observation of two other young children, one of them a boy, with especial reference to the development of the sense of their own relation to the persons who moved about them.

We find no less than four phases of attitude involved in what afterwards becomes the so-called 'social sense' in the child. We say 'afterwards becomes,' because all of them belong in the 'projective' stage of the child's sense of self, i.e. they all go to furnish data which he afterwards appropriates to himself as 'subject.' These four phases are indescribably subtle and indescribably intermixed in the subjective ensemble of the growing child. So much so that we shall not attempt in all cases to cite actual situations to justify each point: rather, the view we take rests upon innumerable situations, and their differences from one another. Just as one is utterly unable to give examples of his own phases of attitude expressive of the *nuances* of meaning which the actions of others bring out of him, so entirely a matter of insight and intuition must his sense be of what is in the child's mind in the various social situations which confront him from day to day. Nevertheless, the drift of the infant's development is very clear to the sympathetic observer; and we think the instances which we cite will be sufficient to excite in all those familiar with little children a sense of the truth of the general portrayal.

I. The first thing in the environment of the infant which it notes — apart from the ordinary fixed and static stimulations, such as sounds, lights, etc. — are *movements*. The first attempts of the infant at anything like steady attention are directed to moving things — a swaying curtain, a moving light, a stroking touch, etc. And further than this, the moving things soon become more than objects of curiosity; these things are just the things that affect him for pleasure or pain. It is movement that brings him his food, movement that regulates the stages of his bath, movement that dresses him comfortably, movement that sings to him and rocks him to sleep. In that complex of sensations, the nurse, the feature of moment to him, of immediate satisfaction, or redemption from pain, is this: movements come to succour him. Change in his bodily feeling is the vital requirement of his life, for by it the rhythm of his vegetative existence is secured; and these changes are accompanied and secured always in the moving presence of the one he sees and feels about him. This, we take it, is the first and great association of the infant with other persons, the earliest reflection in his consciousness of the world of personalities about him. At this stage his 'personality-suggestion' is this *pain-movement-pleasure* psychosis: to this he reacts with a smile, and a crow, and a kick.

Many facts tend to bear us out in this position. My child cried when we handled her in the dark, although we imitated the nurse's movements as closely as possible. She tolerated a strange presence as long as it remained quietly in its place: but let it move, and especially let it usurp any of the pieces of movement-business of the nurse or mother, and her protests were emphatic. The movements tended to bring the strange elements of a new face into the vital association, pain-movement-pleasure, and so to disturb its familiar course: this constituted it a strange 'personality.'

It is astonishing, also, what new accidental elements may become parts of this association. Part of a movement, a gesture, a peculiar habit of the nurse, may become sufficient to give assurance of the welcome presence and the pleasures which the presence brings. Two notes of my song in the night stood for my presence to H., and no song from any one else could replace it. A lighted match stopped the crying of E. for food, although it was but a signal for a process of food-preparation lasting several minutes: and a simple light never stopped her crying under any other circumstances. So with this first start in the sense of personality we find also reasons for the differences of different personalities; but this constitutes the next phase.

2. It is evident that the sense of another's presence thus felt in the infant's consciousness rests, as all associations rest? upon *regularity* or repetition: his sense of expectancy is aroused whenever the chain of events is started. And this is embodied at this stage largely in two indications: the face and the voice. But it is easy to see that this is a very meagre sense of personality; a moving machine which brought pain and alleviated suffering would serve as well. So the child begins to learn in addition the fact that persons are in a measure individual in their treatment of him, and hence that personality has elements of uncertainty or *irregularity* about it. This growing sense is very clear to one who watches an infant in its second half-year. Sometimes its mother gives a biscuit, but sometimes she does not. Sometimes the father smiles and tosses the child; sometimes he does not. And the child looks for signs of these varying moods and methods of treatment. Its new pains of disappointment arise directly on the basis of that former sense of regular personal presence upon which its expectancy went forth.

This new element of the child's 'social sense' becomes, at one period of its development, quite the controlling element. Its action in the presence of the persons of the household becomes hesitating and watchful. Especially does it watch the face for any expressive indications of what treatment is to be expected; for facial expression is now the most regular as well as the most delicate indication. It is unable to anticipate the treatment in detail, and it has not of course learned any principles of interpretation of the conduct of mother or father lying deeper than the details. It is just here, we think, that imitation arises, as will appear later, and becomes so important in the child's life. This is imitation's opportunity. The infant waits to see how others act? because its own weal and woe depends upon this 'how'; and inasmuch as it knows not what to anticipate, its mind is open to every suggestion of movement. Its attention dwells upon details, and by the regular principle of motor reaction which imitation expresses, it acts these suggestions out.

All through the child's second year, and longer, his sense of the persons around him is in this stage. The incessant 'why?' with which he greets any action affecting him, or any information given him, is witness to the simple puzzle of the apparent capriciousness of persons. Of course he cannot understand 'why': so the simple fact to him is that mamma will or won't, he knows not beforehand which.

But in all this period there is germinating in his consciousness — and this very uncertainty is an important element of it — the seed of a far-reaching thought. His sense of persons — moving, pleasure-or-pain-giving, uncertain but self-directing, persons — is now to become a sense of *agency*, of power, which is yet not the power of the regular-moving door on its hinges or the rhythmic swinging of the pendulum of the clock. The sense of personal actuation, 'projective agency,' is now forming, and it again is potent for still further development of the social consciousness. For he begins to grow capricious himself, and to feel that he can be so whenever he likes. Suggestion begins to lose the regularity of its working; or to become negative and 'contrary' in its effects. At this period it is that obedience begins to grow hard, and its meaning begins to dawn upon the child as the great reality. It means the subjection of his own agency, his own liberty to be capricious, to the agency and liberty of some one else.

3. With all this, the child's distinction between and among

the persons who constantly come into contact with him grows on apace? in spite of the element of irregularity of the general fact of personality. As before he learned the difference between one presence and another, — a difference which was overcome in the discovery that every presence is of irregular value; so now he learns the difference between one *character* and another — the regularity of personal agency, as opposed to the regularity of mere associations of movement and to the irregularity of the apparently capricious. Every character is more or less regular in its irregularity. It has its tastes and modes of action, its temperament and type of command. This the child learns late in the second year and thereafter. He behaves differently when the father is in the room. He is quick to obey one person, slow to obey another. He cries aloud, pulls his companions, and behaves reprehensibly generally, when no adult is present but his nurse, who has no authority to punish him. This stage in his 'knowledge of man' leads to those active differences of conduct on his part which make imitation, and the discipline of obedience, a sword with two edges, one for good and one for evil. This general appreciation of character, together with the full-blown social feeling, which constitutes the fourth phase in my division, may be left for later discussion, as well as the part played by this kind of suggestion in the genesis of the moral sense.

To sum up: 'personality-suggestion' is the general term for the stimulations to activity which the child gets from persons. It develops through three or four roughly distinguished 'stages,' all of which illustrate what we have called his 'projective' sense of personality; namely, I. a bare distinction, on the ground of peculiar pain-movement-pleasure complexes, of *persons from things*; 2. a sense of the irregularity or capriciousness of the behaviour of these persons, which is the germ of his *sense of agency*, as opposed to the regular causal series of conditions which things go through; 3. his distinction, vaguely felt but reacted to with great exactness, between the characteristic modes of behaviour or *personal character* of different persons; 4. after his sense of his own subject-agency arises by a process of imitation, he gets what is really *social feeling*: the sense of others as 'ejective,' that is, as like and equal to himself.

III. Deliberative Suggestion — By 'deliberative suggestion' we mean a state of mind in which co-ordinate sense-stimuli meet, confront, oppose, further, one another. Yet we do not mean 'deliberation' in the full-blown volitional sense, but suggestion that appears deliberative, while still inside the reactive consciousness and still representing a single reaction upon a single state of consciousness. In real deliberation, as appears below, there are two or more pictured alternatives, upon the conscious co-ordination of which action follows. But here the different elements are ingredients in a single sensory complex, — one suggestion, — and the motor reaction waits upon the issue of the whole. The competition of processes is probably in large measure subcortical. So the state is still to be classed as sensori-motor, not ideo-motor, since it does not require intelligent memory and representation. The last three months of the child's first year are, we think, clearly given over to this kind of consciousness. Motor stimulations have multiplied, the emotional life is budding forth in a variety of promising traits, the material of conscious character is present but the 'ribs' of mental structure may still be seen through, response answering to appeal in a complex but yet mechanical way. The child lacks self-consciousness, self-decision, self in any developed form.

As an illustration of what we mean, we may record the following case of deliberative suggestion from H.'s thirteenth month: it was more instructive to me than whole books would be on the theory of the conflict of impulses. When about eight months old, H. formed the peculiar habit of suddenly scratching the face of her nurse or mother with her nails. It became fixed in her memory, probably because of the unusual facial expression of pain, reproof, etc., which followed it, until the close proximity of any one's face was sufficient suggestion to her to give it a violent scratch. In order to break up this habit, I began to punish her by taking at once the hand with which she scratched and 'snapping' her fingers with my own first finger hard enough to be painful. For about four weeks this seemed to have no effect, probably because I only saw her a small part of the tune, and only then did she suffer the punishment. But I then observed, and those who were with her most reported, that she only scratched once at a time, and grew very solemn and quiet for some moments afterwards, as if thinking deeply; and soon after this climax was reached she would scratch once impulsively, be punished, and weep profusely, then become as grave as a deacon, looking me in the face. I would then deliberately put my cheek very close to her, and she would sit gazing at it in 'deep thought' for two or even three minutes, hardly moving a muscle the whole time, and then either suddenly scratch my face and be punished again, or turn to something (noise, object, watch chain, etc.) which I was careful enough to provide in Qnier to aid her by drawing off the attention. Having scratched, she began to cry, in anticipation of the punishment. Gradually the scratching became more rare. She seldom yielded to the temptation after being punished, and so the habit entirely disappeared. I may add that her mother and myself endeavoured to induce a different reaction by taking the child's other hand and with it stroking the face which she had scratched. This movement in time replaced the other completely, and the soft stroking became one of her most spontaneous expressions of affection.

Now the first act of scratching was probably accidental, one of the spontaneous reactions or physiological suggestions so common with an infant's hands; it passed, by reason of its peculiar associations, into a sensori-motor reaction whenever the presence of a face acted as suggestion, — so far a strong direct stimulus to the motor centres. Then came the pain of punishment, — a stimulus to the inhibition on the next occasion, not by exciting a clear memory, but by working itself directly into the suggesting psychosis, and thus reducing the motor tendency. For a time the tendency remained strong enough, however, to cause the reaction; then there followed an apparent balance between the two, and finally the pain element predominated in the suggestion, and the reaction was permanently inhibited. The stroking reaction gained all the strength of violent and repeated association with the elements of this mental conflict, and was thus soon fixed and permanent.

Taking this as a typical case of 'deliberative suggestion,' — and I could instance many others from H.'s life history and from E.'s, — two inferences may be brought out in passing: *there is nothing here that requires volition*, meaning by 'volition' a new influence of any kind, — active consciousness; if we do call it so, we simply apply a different term to phenomena which in their simplicity we call by other names. And, second, *suggestion is as original a motor stimulus as pleasure and pain*. Here they are in direct conflict. Can we say that H. balanced the pleasure of scratching and the pain of punishment, and decided the case on this egoistic basis? What pleasure did the scratching have more than any other muscular exercise? It was simply a sensori-motor habit which the pain inhibition tended to break up.

So also, apart from pathological *aboulia*, which is described later on, we find a corresponding condition in adult life. As I have said elsewhere, "there is a state of conflict and hindrance among presentations which is mechanical in its issue, . . . so states of vexation, divided counsel, conflicting impulse, and hasty decision against one's desire for deliberate choice. We often find ourselves drawn violently apart, precipitated through a whirl of suggested courses into a course which we feel unwilling to acknowledge as our own." Many of the conditions of deliberation are there, but not the fact of it.

Ideo-motor Suggestion

By ideo-motor suggestion I mean the condition in which the stimulus is a clearly pictured idea, a presentation or object with all its 'meaning,' or a revived image of memory or imagination.

Imitation — For a long period after the child has learned to use all his senses' and after his memory is well developed, he lacks conscious imitation entirely. I have been quite unable with my children to confirm the results of Preyer, who attributes imitation to his child at the age of three to four months.

In support of the assertion that imitation is rather late in its rise, the following experiences may be reported. As a necessary caution, the rule was made that no single performance should be considered real imitation unless it could be brought out again under similar circumstances. This rule is necessary, I think, merely for caution, since the 'copy' set for imitation is likely to be some simple movement of lips, hands, etc., which the child has made himself before, and is likely to make again. It is possible also from the mere fact of dynamogeny that the motor discharge in shedding itself outward would tend in a general way to find its most permeable native pathway toward the muscles which repeat the copy, since the movements are natural and easy. At any rate, such cases, if they exist, shade up gradually into conscious imitations.

It is probable, therefore, that cases of imitation recorded as happening as early as the third month are merely coincidences. For example, I recorded an apparent imitation by H., of closing the hand, as late as May 22 (beginning of the ninth month), but afterwards I wrote, " experiment not confirmed with repeated trials running through four succeeding days." H.'s first clear imitation was on May 24, in knocking a bunch of keys against a vase, as she saw me do it, in order to produce the bell-like sound. This she repeated over and over again, and tried to reproduce it a week later, when, from lapse of time, she had partly forgotten how to use the keys. But on the same day, May 24, other efforts to bring out imitation failed signally, i.e. with more or less articulate sounds, movements of the lips (Preyer's experiments), and opening and closing of the hands. Ten days later, however, she imitated closing the hand on three different occasions. And a week afterward she imitated movements of the lips and certain sounds, as *pa, ma,* etc. From this time forward the phenomenon seemed extended to a very wide range of activities, and began to assume the immense importance which it always comes to have in the life of the young child.

When the imitative impulse does come, it comes in earnest. For many months after its rise it may be called, perhaps, the controlling impulse, apart from the ordinary life processes. As a phenomenon, it is too familiar to need description. Its importance in the growth of the child's mind is largely in connection with the development of language and of voluntary movement generally.

The phenomena may be divided into two general classes, called *simple imitation* and *persistent imitation.'* By 'simple' imitations, reactions are characterized, in which the movement does not imitate well, but is the best the child can do. He does not try to improve by making a second attempt. This is evidently a case of simple sensori-motor suggestion, and is peculiar psychologically only because of the more or less remote approximation the reaction has to the model that the child copies.

Surveying the ground that we have gone over so far in this chapter, the progress of suggestion may be seen by the following brief definitions: —

1. *Physiological suggestion* is the tendency of a reflex or secondary automatic process to get itself associated with and influenced by stimulating processes of a physiological and vaguely sensory sort. Perhaps the plainest case of it, on a large scale in animal life, is seen in the decay of instincts when no longer suited to the creature's needs and environment.

2. *Sensori-motor and ideo-motor suggestion* is the tendency of all nervous reactions to adapt themselves to new stimulations, both sensory and ideal, in such a way as to be more ready for the repetition or continuance of these stimulations.

3. *Deliberative suggestion* is the tendency of different competing sensory processes to merge in a single conscious state with a single motor reaction, illustrating the principles of nervous summation and arrest.

4. *Imitative suggestion* is the tendency of a sensory or ideal process to maintain itself by such an adaptation of its discharges that they reinstate in turn new stimulations of the same kind.

Whether any simpler formulation of these partial statements may be reached, is a question which may be delayed until we have looked more closely at certain other instances of suggestion, which have not been described before, and at the conditions of nervous adaptation in general.

Subconscious Adult Suggestion

There are certain phenomena of a rather striking kind coming under this head whose classification is so evident that discussion of the general psychological principles which they involve is not necessary. The kind of fact which I have in view may be illustrated with sufficient clearness merely by the recital of the following observations.

Tune-suggestion. — Professor Ladd has pointed out in de- tail — what has for a long time been taken for granted — that dream states are largely indebted for their visual elements, what we see in our dreams, to accidental lines, patches, etc., in the field of vision, when the eyes are shut, due to the distended blood vessels of the cornea and lids, to changes in the external illumination, to the presence of dust particles of different configuration, etc. The other senses also undoubtedly contribute to the texture of our dreams by equally subconscious suggestions. And there is no doubt, further, that our waking life is constantly influenced by equally trivial stimulations.

Often, when a tune springs up 'in my head,' the same tune has been lately sung or whistled in my hearing, though quite unconsciously to myself. Often the tunes are those heard in church the previous day or earlier. Such a tune I am entirely unable to recall voluntarily: yet when it comes into my mind's ear, so to speak, I readily recognize it as belonging to an earlier day's experience. Other cases show various accidental suggestions, such as the tune 'Mozart' suggested by the composer's name, the tune 'Gentle Annie' suggested by the name Annie, etc. In all these cases it is only after the tune has taken possession of consciousness, and after much seeking, that the suggesting influence is discovered.

Closer analysis reveals the following facts. The 'time' of such internal tunes is usually dictated by some rhythmical subconscious occurrence. After hearty meals it is always the time of the heart-beat, unless there be 'in the air' some more impressive stimulus; as, for example, when on shipboard, the beat is with me invariably that of the engine throbs. When walking it is the rhythm of the foot-fall. On one occasion a knock of four beats on the door started the Marseillaise in my ear: following up this clue, I found that at any time, different divisions of musical time being struck on the table at will by another person, tunes would spring up and run on, getting their cue from the measures suggested. Further, when a tune dies away, its last notes often suggest, some time after, another having a similar movement — just as we pass from one tune to another in a 'medley.' It may also be noted that in my case the tune memories are *auditive*: they run in my head when I have no words for them and have never sung them — an experience which is consistent with the fact that these 'internal tunes' arise in childhood before the faculty of speech.

Dreams as Emotion Stimulus. — Another important realm of suggestion, not hitherto explored, is seen in the influence of dreams on the waking life. Dreams react to deepen waking impressions, and to strengthen the hold of dominant presentations and impulses. This fact seems to have its primary application to emotion. We cannot tell how much of the active momentum of our waking life we owe to dream stimulation. The following case of fact, in the life of my little girl H., indicates that such a stimulus may be of enormous importance. When two years and three months of age, she was accidentally run over by a dog. Before this she had been very fond of dogs. She was not much hurt, but very much frightened, and repeated to every one the words, 'Doggie run over baby.' The next day she saw a dog on the street and showed some signs of fear until the brute ran away. About the second night after the occurrence her mother and I were awakened by a violent outcry in H.'s room. On going in, the child was found sitting in bed undergoing a paroxysm of fear from a bad dream. She repeated again and again after leaving the room, 'Doggie run over baby ana' (ana was her word for *there*), pointing into her bedroom. Evidently she had lived over again in her dream the occurrence with the dog. The effect on her waking life was very marked. The next day she could not be induced to go into her bedroom, protesting, 'Doggie in ana,' and crying lustily if the endeavour wa.s made to carry her. Further, for several days the sight of a dog on the street threw her into such convulsive fits of fear that her nurse brought her home to be quieted — a much more violent exhibition, be it noted, than that which occurred after the real occurrence with the dog, but before the dream. The sight or even the picture of a dog long excited great emotion, and it is not unlikely that she will carry for life this antipathy, which will appear later to be unaccountable.

Normal Auto-suggestion. — A further class of suggestions, which fall under the general phrase 'auto-suggestion,' of a normal type, may be illustrated. In experimenting upon the possibility of suggesting sleep to another, we have found certain strong reactive influences upon our own mental condition. Such an effort, which involves the picturing of another as asleep, is a strong auto-suggestion of sleep, taking effect in my own case in about five minutes if the conditions be kept constant. The more clearly the patient's sleep is pictured, the stronger becomes the subjective feeling of drowsiness. After about ten minutes the ability to give strong concentration seems to disintegrate, attention is renewed only by fits and starts and in the presence of great mental inertia, and the oncoming of sleep is almost overpowering. A frequent cure for insomnia, speaking for myself, is the persistent effort to put some one else asleep by hard thinking of the end in view, with a continued gentle movement, such as stroking the other with the hand.

On the other hand, it is impossible to bring on a state of drowsiness by imagining myself asleep. The first effort at this, indeed, is promising, for it leads to a state of restfulness and ease akin to the mental composure which is the usual prelimunary to sleep; but it goes no farther. It is succeeded by a state of steady wakefulness, which effort of attention or effort not to attend only intensifies. If the victim of insomnia could only forget that he is thus afflicted, could forget himself altogether, his case would be more hopeful. The contrast between this condition and that already described shows that it is the self-idea, with the emotions it awakens, which prevents the suggestion from realizing itself and probably accounts for many cases of insomnia.

The attempt to analyze out the emotional 'moments' which enter into the latter case yields some such result as the following. It is impossible to think of self, however vaguely and fugitively, without inducing positive emotional excitement. All the intense self-motives which practical life keeps alive — the most vigorous expressive influences of our mental nature — at once tend to spring up from their nascent state. There are really no proper distinctions among them: pride shades down to complacency, complacency merges into mild interest, interest becomes intensified in anxiety or fear. Or the mere thought of self starts a train of affairs through consciousness about which personal concern is lively. When one thinks of himself, a kind of egoistic excitement at once arises. It is undoubtedly these subjective elements, these emotional phases, which prevent such conscious auto-suggestions from realizing themselves.

Sense Exaltation — Recent hypnotic discussions have shown the remarkable exaltation which the senses may attain in somnambulism, together with a corresponding refinement in the interpretative faculty. Events, etc., quite subconscious, usually become suggestions of direct influence upon the subject. Unintended gestures, habitual with the experimenter, may suffice to hypnotize his accustomed subject. The possibility of such training of the senses in the normal state has not had sufficient emphasis. The young child's subtle discriminations of facial and other personal indications are remarkable. The prolonged experience of putting H. to sleep — extending over a period of more than six months, during which I slept beside her bed — served to make me alive to a certain class of suggestions otherwise quite beyond notice.

In the first place, we may note the intense auto-suggestion of sleep already pointed out, under the stimulus of repeated nursery rhymes regularly resorted to in putting the child asleep. Second, surprising progressive exaltation of hearing and the interpretation of sounds coming from her in a dark room. At the end of four or five months, her movements in bed awoke me or not according as she herself was awake or not.

Again, the same phenomenon to an equally marked degree attended the sound of her breathing. It is well enough known that the smallest functional bodily change induces changes in both the rapidity and the quality of the respiration. [8] In sleep the muscles of inhalation and exhalation are relaxed, inhalation becomes long and deep, exhalation short and exhaustive, and the rhythmic intervals of respiration much lengthened. Now degrees of relative wakefulness are indicated with surprising delicacy by the slight respiration sounds given forth by the sleeper. Professional nurses learn to interpret these indications with great skill. This kind of hearing-exaltation became very pronounced in my operations with my child. After some experience the peculiar breathing of advancing or actual wakefulness in the child was sufficient to wake me. And when awake myself, the change in the infant's respiration-sounds to those indicative of oncoming sleep was sufficient to suggest or bring on sleep in myself. In the dark, also, the general character of her breathing-sounds was interpreted with great accuracy in terms of her varied needs, her comfort or discomfort, etc. The same kind of suggestion from the respiration-sounds now troubles me whenever any one is sleeping within hearing distance

The reactions in movement upon these suggestions are very marked and appropriate, in customary or habitual lines, although the stimulations are quite subconscious. The clearest illustrations in this body of my experiences were afforded by my responses in crude songs to the infant's waking movements and breathing-sounds. I have often waked myself by myself singing one of two nursery rhymes, which by endless repetition night after night had become so automatic as to follow in a reactive way upon the sense-stimulus from the child. It is certainly astonishing that among the things which one may get to do automatically, we find automatic singing: but writers on mental defect have noted that the function of musical or semi-musical expression may be reflex.

The principle of subconscious suggestion, of which these simple facts are less important illustrations, has very interesting applications in the higher reaches of social, moral, and educational theory. I have applied the phrase 'plastic imitation' to certain of the social and educational phenomena.

Inhibitory Suggestion

An interesting class of phenomena which figure perhaps at all the levels of suggestion now described, may be known as 'inhibitory suggestions.' The phrase, in its broadest use, refers to all cases in which the suggesting stimulus tends to suppress, check, inhibit, movement. We find this in certain cases just as strongly marked as the positive movementbringing kind of suggestion. The facts may be put under certain heads in relation to the types of suggestion already enumerated, the general theory being left over for the doctrine of mental development found in subsequent chapters.

Pain Suggestion — Of course, the fact that pain inhibits movement occurs at once to the reader. As far as this is true always, and is a native inherited thing, it is organic, and so falls under the head of 'physiological suggestion' of a negative sort. The child shows contracting movements, crying movements, starting and jumping movements, shortly after birth, and so plainly that we need not hesitate to say that these pain responses are provided for in his nervous system; and that, in general, they are inhibitory and contrary to those other native reactions which indicate pleasure. Our theory provides, as stated below, a way of accounting for this state of things.

The influence of pain, besides being thus a physiological datum, extends everywhere through mental development. It is one of our main objects to try to ascertain its exact function, both in individual and in race development; so any further word upon it here would only anticipate later detailed treatment. The general fact, however, is this: that pain suggests a lively muscular revolt away from every stimulus which produces it; and this statement includes, of course, the inhibition of any movement which brings pain, since this movement is itself felt as a stimulating or incoming process along those afferent nerve courses which serve as the apparatus of the muscular sense.

Control Suggestion — This covers all cases which show any kind of restraint set upon the movements of the body short of that which comes from voluntary intention. The infant brings the movements of his legs, arms, head, etc., gradually into some kind of order and system. This is accomplished by a system of orgamc checks and counterchecks, by which associations are formed between muscular sensations and certain other sensations, as of sight, touch, hearing, etc. The latter serve as suggestions to the performance of those movements, and those only, which produce the former. The infant learns to hold up his head, to raise his trunk, to extend his hands, to grasp with thumb opposite the four fingersCall purely by such control suggestions.

These cases come so near to the sphere of voluntary action — indeed, they pass so directly into volitions — that they are more profitably discussed in the chapter devoted to that topic. We will there see reasons for rejecting the view of some, that these are voluntary acts on the part of the child. The few new observations which I have to offer on this topic may also be reserved.

Contrary Suggestion — By this is meant a tendency of a very singular kind observable in many children, no less than in many adults, to do the contrary when any course is suggested. The very word 'contrary' is used in popular talk to describe an individual who shows this type of conduct. Such a child or man is rebellious whenever rebellion is possible; he seems to kick constitutionally against the pricks. My child E. showed it in her second year in a very marked way. When told that a new taste was 'good' — a suggestion readily taken in its positive sense by her sister at that age — she would turn away with a show of distaste even when she had liked the same taste earlier. When asked to give her hand into mine, — a case of direct imitative suggestion, — she thrust it behind her back. The sight of hat and cloak was a signal for a tempest, although she enjoyed outdoor excursions. These are only instances from many of her contrary suggestions at this period. The tendency yielded to the all-conquering onset of imitation late in her second year, and she is now (third year) as docile an imitator as one could desire.

The fact of 'contrariness' in older children — especially boys — is so familiar to all who have observed school children with any care, that I need not cite further details. And men and women often become so enslaved to suggestions of contrary that they seem only to wait for indications of the wishes of others in order to oppose and thwart them.

Contrary suggestions are to be explained as exaggerated instances of control. It is easy to see that the checks and counter-checks already spoken of as constituting the method of suggestive control of movement — that these may themselves become so habitual and intense as to dominate the reactions which they should only regulate. The associations between the muscular series and the visual series, let us say, which controls it, comes to work backwards, so that the drift of the organic processes is toward certain contrary reverse movements. Certain of the other associates of the control series also, especially those which, by strong contrasting experiences of pleasure and pain, represent in any sense a contrary series, may become dominating. While in the case of simple movements, as I have said, the dominant associates are only the same motor and visual series read backwards; yet the range of contrast effects secured by association extends to all cases of opposing systems of movement and suggestions of conduct. So contrary suggestion becomes clear as a case of auto-suggestion in which the stimulating sensation or thought is itself started up in sharp contrast and habitual opposition to a present external suggestion of the regular kind.

In the higher reaches of conduct and life we find interesting cases of very refined contrary suggestion. In the man of ascetic temperament, the duty of self-denial takes the form of a regular contrary suggestion in opposition to every invitation to self-indulgence, however innocent. And the overscrupulous mind, like the over-precise, is a prey to the eternal remonstrances from the contrary which intrude their advice into all his decisions. In matters of thought and belief, also, cases are common of stubborn opposition to evidence, and persistence in opinion, which are in no way due to the cogency of the contrary argument, or to real force of conviction.

Bashfulness — I may first report observations on this interesting fact of child-life, considered as an exhibition of what has been called 'inhibitory suggestion'; and then show its bearings.

The general character of a child's bashfulness need not be enlarged upon. Its form of expression is also familiar. It begins to appear generally in the first year, showing itself as an inhibiting influence upon the child's normal activities. Its most evident signs are nervous fingerings of dress, objects, hands, etc., turning away of head and body, bowing of head and hiding of face, awkward movements of trunk and legs, and in extreme cases, reddening of the face, puckering of lips and eye muscles, and finally cries and weeping. An important difference, however, is observable in these exhibitions according as the child is accompanied by a familiar person or not. When the mother or nurse is present, many of the signs seem to be useful in securing concealment from the eye of strangers — behind dress or apron or figure of the familiar person. In the absence, however, of such a refuge the child sinks often into a state of general passivity or inhibition of movement, akin to the sort of paralysis usually associated with great fear.

This analogy with the physical signs of fear gives a real indication, I think, of the race origin of bashfulness, which is probably a differentiation of fear. This I cannot dwell upon now, but simply suggest that bashfulness arose as a special utility-reaction on occasion of fear of persons, in view of personal qualities possessed by the one who fears. The concealing tendency also shows the parallel development of intimate personal relationships of protection, support, etc., and so gives indications of certain early social conditions.

I. The child is earliest seized with what may be called

'primary' or 'organic' bashfulness akin to the organic stages in the well-recognized instinctive emotions, such as fear, anger, sympathy, etc. This exhibition occurs in the first year and marks the attitudes of the infant toward strangers. It is not so much inhibitory of action in this first stage; it rather takes on the positive signs of fear, with protestation, shrinking, crying, etc. It falls easily under the type of reaction described as 'sensori-motor suggestion,' above; being very largely provided for in the nervous equipment of the child at this age.

The duration of this stage depends largely upon the child's social environment. The passage from the attitude of instinctive antipathy toward outsiders, and that of affection equally instinctive toward the members of the household, over into a more reasonable sense of the difference between proved friends and unproved strangersCthis depends directly upon the growth of the sense of general social relationships established by experience. One of the most important elements in the child's progress' in this way' out of its 'organic' social life, is the degree and variety of its intercourse with other children, and indeed also with other adults, than those of its own home. Children carried to summer hotels every year, or brought frequently into the drawing-room to see the mothers' callers, soon lose all 'fear of strangers' and become quite frankly approachable, even showing great liking for society at the tender age of a year and a half or so. On the other hand, children kept in extreme isolation from strangers, young or old, may show extraordinary paralysis of all motor functions, of a markedly organic kind, steadily for two or three years later on in their development, when brought suddenly into the presence of those who are unfamiliar.

The rapidity with which a child gets over its organic bashfulness varies also remarkably with the attitudes of older children whom he sees. Nothing else cures a child of this physical shyness as quickly as the example of an older child. This is also one of the marked offices of imitation. It presents to the imitative child an example or 'copy,' which tends to bring out his action in definite ways earlier than his own organic growth would in itself have warranted. The child by instinct imitates movements, etc., which he would otherwise have waited to acquire largely by accident. In this way the stages of social growth are very materially shortened.

2. We find next a period of strong social tendency in the child, of toleration of strangers and liking for persons generally, in great contrast to the attitudes of organic distrust of the earlier period just mentioned. There seems to be in this a reaction against the instinct of social self-preservation characteristic of the earlier stage. It is due in all likelihood to the actual experience of the child in receiving kind treatment from strangers — kinder in the way of indiscriminate indulgence than the more orderly treatment which it gets from its own parents. Everybody comes to be trusted on first acquaintance by the child, through the teachings of his own experience, just as in the earlier years everybody was treated by him, under the instincts of his inherited nature, as an agent of possible harm. That this new phase of social attitude is learned from experience is seen in the absence of this confidence, on the part of the child, toward animals. The fear, purely of the organic stage, persists in the child's thoughts of animals which are new to him, and only becomes more confirmed as he fails to get the same reasons for 'modifying his opinion' that teach him to tolerate strange persons more and more comfortably. The contrast is strongly brought out sometimes when such a young child meets animals in public places. He then turns to persons for protection, even to the strange persons before whom, under ordinary circumstances, he would stand abashed. His native sense of social protection, at first limited to his natural protectors in his own house, has come to extend to all persons, as against such common enemies

as the brutes.

3. Finally we note the return of bashfulness in the child's third year and later. This time it is bashfulness in the proper sense of the term, rid of the element of fear, and rid, largely, of its compelling organic force and methods of expression. The bashful five-year-old smiles in the midst of his hesitations, draws near to the object of his curiosity, is evidently overwhelmed with the sense of his own presence rather than with that of his new acquaintance, and indulges in actions calculated to *keep notice drawn to himself.*

The reality of this group of the child's social attitudes, and the great contrast which they present to those of the organic period, can hardly have too much emphasis. It is one of the great outstanding facts of his progressive relation to the elements of his social *milieu.* There is a sort of self-exhibition, almost of coquetry, in the child's behaviour; which shows the most remarkable commingling of native organic elements with the social lessons of personal well- and ill-desert which are now becoming of such importance in his life. All this makes so marked a contrast to the exhibitions of organic bashfulness that it constitutes in my opinion a most important resource for the study of the evolution of the social sense.

In this last case we have before us, in short, a phenomenon of rather complex self-consciousness — a thing of ideal value — and its suggestion-complexes, as they body themselves forth in the child's reactions, tell of his extraordinary progress in the understanding of himself and the world. He now begins to show the germ of modesty and of all the emotions akin to and contrary to it.

With this degree of progress we may now leave the child, not undertaking the discussion of the development of true modesty in its later stages in the intricate special movements of adolescence: but it remains to point out the congruity between this scheme of the child's different behaviours in respect to persons and the different personal suggestions which in an earlier place we found him actually getting from others.

It will be remembered that several aspects of the child's personal environment were found to appeal to him in a progressive way. It seemed fair to think that persons are at first to him only a peculiar part of his 'projected" presented, objective, world of things. He has 'personal projects,, as we found it well to call them' before he has any sense of himself as a spiritual being or as the subject of his own mental processes. The getting of objects seems to be part of the business for which his nervous equipment more or less adequately provides, and among these objects, the persons who move around him get themselves characterized by very important marks.

The observation of organic bashfulness tends' when viewed in connection with this earlier point, to confirm this view of the way the child begins to apprehend persons; and at the same time, it enables us to see a little farther. For strange as it may appear' we are here confronted with an element of organic equipment especially fitted to receive and respond to these peculiar objects, persons' 'personal projects., The child strikes instinctively an extraordinary series of attitudes when persons appear among his objects' attitudes which other objects, *qua* objects, do not excite. And later in life' in the organic effects indicative of modesty, such as blushing, hesitating, etc.' we find similar signs of a social *rapport* which has grown into the very fibres of our nerves. These attitudes extend somewhat to animals, as we have seen; and that makes it all the more striking. For animals are persons, to a child of that age; they act upon him through his animal parts, through physical pains, pleasures, fears, etc., and that is the only way that persons also can act upon an infant a year old.

We have to say, therefore, that the child is born to be a member of society, in the same sense, precisely, that he is born with eyes and ears to see and hear the movements and sounds of the world, and with touch to feel the things of space; and, as I hope to show later in detail? all views of the man as a total creature, a creation, must recognize him not as a single soul shut up in a single body to act, or to abstain from acting' upon others similarly shut up in similar bodies; but as a soul partly in his own body, partly in the bodies of others, to all intents and purposes, so intimate is this social bond a service for which he pays in kind, since we see in his body, considered simply as a physical organism, preparation for the reception of the soul-life, the suggestions of mind and spirit, of those others. I do not see wherein the community of the senses together, in a single life of nervous activity, differs very much in conception from this community of men, bound together by the native ties which lie at the basis of their most abstract and developed social organizations.

Again, the second phase of the child's actions in the presence of persons — the freer, more ready reception of strangers and intercourse with them' seen usually during the second year — this also gives us what our earlier notes on 'personality-suggestion' would lead us to expect. We saw that the child begins to find out more about persons, and so to gain associations which give him the beginning of certain expectations regarding them; self-formed expectations, that is, no longer dependent merely upon the stirrings of instinct and inherited impulse. He learns that pleasure almost always comes from persons, and so does the alleviation of pain. This is a mortal blow at organic bashfulness, as every father and mother knows. A lump of sugar will very soon release the inhibitions of the shy year-old. Then he further learns something of the characteristics of persons, the irregularity of personal action, the presence of the 'personal equation' of mood and feeling in those nearest to him. This leads him to seek out methods, somewhat individual to himself, of pleasing these near persons and of securing their smile and approbation, or of escaping the reproofs which even his shyness brings; and these he substitutes for the blinder attempt, which nature taught him, to hide his physical person.

And he also learns our habits, the regularities of character in adults, and so learns that nobody means to hurt him, after all. It is amusing how soon a two- or three-year-old child 'sizes up' a stranger, and meets him halfway with conduct more or less appropriately attuned to the indications of character shown in the face and acts of the newcomer.

So, with all this, the instinctive or 'organic' bashfulness gets rapidly rubbed away. But it is now clear that the means of this freedom from it are all social. A child's growth away from the instinct of social fear to the apprehension of social truth, and all his actions midway in this progress, come only from varied and persistent experience of people and appeals to living examples. How can character be apprehended if characters are absent? And how can character schemes be grown into, if the regularity of the child's life is of so narrow a scope that all the threads of his social relationship run the same way, and no tangles and confusions arise to bring out his own strenuous action and his rebellions against his native reflex ways of behaviour?

The oncoming of true bashfulness, finally, — the bashfulness which shows reflection, in its simpler form, upon self and the actions of self, — represents the child's direct application of what he knows of persons to his own inner life. It is what we have called the 'subjective' stage in his sense of personality.

But, as we shall also see, this grows only apace with the contrary movement by which he assigns his own enriched mental experience back to his teacher, and seeks his further judgment upon it. The child, when he knows himself able to draw a figure, for example, does not know this alone, or this completely. He has also the sense of the social 'copy' or example from which the lesson was learned, and further and with it, he knows that his performance is again subject to revision in light of the approval or disapproval of teacher or friend. The performances of the self cannot in any case be freed from the sense of possible inspection by others, and the child shrinks from this inspection. This has further development below. Suffice it to say that in this higher *rapport,* which involves clearly the sense of self-agency, but self-agency still tied down to the agency of other people like self, — here in the real reflective relation of self to others, — comes the third and crowning stage of the class of phenomena known by the word 'bashfulness.' My children do their imperfect tasks for me because they know me to understand and be indulgent: even the elder assumes the patron, and says of the younger: 'She is so little, you know.' But in the presence of the stranger whose opinion is not known beforehand, they are bashful with the sense of new standards perhaps firmly insisted upon. This is where the inhibiting suggestion of true bashfulness appears: that of modesty, and clearly also that of certain ethical emotions.

The whole situation becomes, I may add, an extraordinary point of vantage for estimating the development view of the origin of the social and personal sense. We have in it direct evidence of the growth of the social instinct by accretions from experiences of social conditions — or if we go into refinements of biological theory, from the adding up of variations all fitted to survive socially — and direct evidence, further? of the lines of progress which these experiences and variations have marked out. For the infant is an embryo person, a social unit in the process of forming; and he is, in these early stages, plainly recapitulating the items in the social history of the race.

This social evolution presents a phase, therefore, of general development in which the theory that the individual goes through stages which repeat the race-stages of his species ought to find illustrations of more than common value. For the social life is a late attainment, whether considered anthropologically or racially, and the child waits to begin the series of 'laps in the social race' until he meets us, his observers, face to face. The embryology of society is open to study in the nursery.

I think, accordingly, that several important hints at the history of societies, both animal and human, are afforded by the phenomena of bashfulness as now described. These I can do no more than mention at present.

Organic bashfulness would seem to represent the instinctive fear shown by the higher animals, coupled with the natural family and gregarious instincts which they have. This shades up into the more fearless and more confiding attitudes of certain passably peaceable creatures, which take kindly to domestication, and depend more upon animal organizations and natural defences, such as those afforded by geographical distribution, coloration, habits of life, etc., for their protection. For the social protections are after all more effective for the defence of racial life and propagation than the special instinctive armament of individuals. Then, of course, only in man do we find the stage of reflective thought on self and the social relations of self, which is seen germinating in the child in the third year or later.

The parallel seems also to be worth something to the anthropologist when he comes to inquire into the history of the human species. Admitting with Westermarck that man as a species is monogamous and tends to family life, we should find in his earliest history the period corresponding to the organic bashfulness of the child; and its instinctive presence in the very young child lends some support, perhaps, to Westermarck's view. The later tribal and nomadic conditions possibly tended to release the cords of an instinct so purely defensive, and to bring in the freer range of peaceful pursuits represented, it is conceivable, by the second stage of the child's history; while again the stage of development of the distinctly industrial, artistic, and commercial life of man, with its social ways of solving all problems of public welfare, corresponds to the more reflective attainments of the period which is seen dawning in the true bashfulness of the three-year-old. For there can be no doubt that recent writers are correct in finding that the more refined egoism is a reflex from the more generalized socialism; a thesis which social psychology takes now from the analyses of men like Balzac and Bourget and the insights of Tarde and the historians of society; but one which it is itself quite able, I think, to make good by its own methods of inquiry.

Hypnotic Suggestion

The facts upon which the current theories of hypnotism are based may be summed up under a few heads, and the recital of them will serve to bring this class of phenomena into the general lines of classification drawn out in this chapter.

The Facts — When by any cause the attention is held fixed upon an object, say a bright button, for a sufficient time without distraction, the subject begins to lose consciousness in a progressive way. Generalizing this simple experiment, we may say that any method or device which serves to secure undivided and prolonged attention to any kind of a 'suggestion,' — be it object, idea, anything that can be thought about, — this brings on what is called hypnosis to a person normally constituted.

The Paris school of interpreters find three stages of progress in the hypnotic sleep: First, *catalepsy,* characterized by rigid fixity of the muscles in any position in which the limbs may be put by the experimenter, with great *suggestibility* on the side of consciousness, and anæsthesia in certain areas of the skin and in certain of the special senses; second, *lethargy,* in which consciousness seems to disappear entirely, the subject cannot be aroused by any sense stimulation by eye, ear, skin, etc., and the body is flabby and pliable as in natural sleep; third, *somnambulism,* so called from its analogies to the ordinary sleep-walking condition to which many persons are subject. This last covers the phenomena of ordinary mesmeric exhibitions at which traveling mesmerists 'control' persons before audiences and make them obey their commands. While other scientists properly deny these distinct stages as such, they may yet be taken as representing extreme instances of the phenomena, and serve as points of departure for further discussion.

On the mental side the general characteristics of hypnotic somnambulism are as follows: I. *The impairing of memory* in a peculiar way: In the hypnotic condition all affairs of the ordinary life are forgotten; on the other hand, after waking, the events of the hypnotic condition are forgotten. Further, in any subsequent period of hypnosis the events of the former similar periods are remembered. So a person who is habitually hypnotized has two continuous memories; one for the events of his normal life, only when he is normal, and one for the events of his hypnotic periods, only when he is hypnotized.

2. Suggestibility to a remarkable degree. By this is meant the tendency of the subject to have in reality any mental condition which is suggested to him. He is subject to

suggestions both on the side of his receptivity to impressions and on the side of action. He will see, hear, remember, believe, refuse to see, hear, etc., anything, with some doubtful exceptions, which may be suggested to him by word or deed, or even by the slightest and perhaps unconscious indications of those about him. On the side of conduct his suggestibility is equally remarkable. Not only will he act in harmony with the illusions of sight, etc., suggested to him, but he will carry out, like an automaton, the actions suggested to him. Further, pain, pleasure, and the organic accompaniments of them may be produced by suggestion. The arm may be actually scarred with a lead-pencil if the patient be told that it is red-hot iron. A suggested pain brings vasomotor and other bodily changes that prove, as similar tests in the other cases prove, that simulation is impossible and the phenomena are real. These phenomena and those given below are no longer based on the mere reports of the 'mesmerists,' but are the recognized property of legitimate psychology.

Again, such suggestions may be for a future time, and get themselves performed only when a determined interval has elapsed; they are then called *deferred* or *post-hypnotic* suggestions. Post-hypnotic suggestions are those which include the command not to perform them until a certain time after the subject has returned to his normal condition; such suggestions are — if of reasonably trifling character — actually carried out afterward in the normal state, although the person is conscious of no reason why he should act in such a way, having no remembrance whatever that he had received the suggestion when hypnotized. Such post-hypnotic performances may be deferred by suggestion for many months.

3. So-called *exaltation* of the mental faculties, especially of the senses: increased acuteness of vision, hearing, touch, memory, and the mental functions generally. By reason of

this great 'exaltation,' hypnotized patients may get suggestions which are not intended, from experimenters, and discover their intentions when every effort is made to conceal them. Often emotional changes in expression are discerned by them; and if it be admitted that their power of logical and imaginative insight is correspondingly exalted, there is practically no limit to the patient's ability to read, simply from physical indications, the mental states of those who experiment with him.

4 So-called *rapport*. This term covers all the facts known, before the subject was scientifically investigated, by such expressions as 'personal magnetism,' 'will power' over the subject, etc. It is true that one particular operator alone may be able to hypnotize a particular patient; and in this case the patient is, when hypnotized, open to suggestions only from this person. He is deaf and blind to everything enjoined by any one else. It is easy to see from what has already been said that this does not involve any occult nerve influence or mental power. A sensitive patient anybody can hypnotize, provided only that the patient have the idea or conviction that the experimenter possesses such power. Now, let a patient get the idea that only one man can hypnotize him, and that is the beginning of the hypnotic suggestion itself. It is a part of the suggestion that a certain personal *rapport* is necessary; so the patient must have this *rapport*. This is shown by the fact that, when such a patient is hypnotized, the operator in *rapport* with him can transfer the so-called control to any one else simply by suggesting to the patient that this third party can also hypnotize him. *Rapport*, therefore, and all the amazing claims of charlatans to powers of charming, stealing another's personality, controlling his will at a distance — all such claims are explained, as far as they have anything to rest upon, by suggestion under conditions of mental hyperaesthesia or exaltation.

I may now add certain practical remarks which may tend to mark off the range of the phenomena more clearly.

In general, any method which fixes the attention to a single stimulus long enough is probably sufficient to produce hypnosis; but the result is quick and profound in proportion as the patient has the idea that it is going to succeed, i.e. gets the suggestion of sleep. It may be said, therefore, that the elaborate performances, such as passes, rubbings, mysterious incantations, etc., often resorted to, have no physiological effect whatever, and only seem to work in the way of suggestion upon the mind of the subject. In view of this it is probable that any person in normal health can be hypnotized, provided he is not too sceptical of the operator's knowledge and powers; and, on the contrary, any one can hypnotize another, provided he do not arouse too great scepticism, and is not himself wavering and clumsy. It is probable, however, that susceptibility varies greatly in degree, and that race exerts an important influence. Thus in Europe the French seem to be the most susceptible, and the English and Scandinavians the least so. The impression that weak-minded persons are most available is quite mistaken. On the contrary, patients in the insane asylums, idiots, etc., are the most refractory. This is to be expected, from the fact that in these cases power of strong. steady attention is wanting. The only one class of pathological cases which seem peculiarly open to the hypnotic influence is that of the hystero-epileptics, whose tendencies are toward extreme suggestibility. Further, one may hypnotize himself — so-called *auto-suggestion* — especially after having been put into the trance more than once by others.

So-called 'criminal suggestions' may be made, with more or less effect, in the hypnotic state. Cases have been tried in the French courts, in which evidence for and against such influence of a third person over the criminal has been admitted. The reality of the phenomenon, however, is in dispute. The

Paris school claims that criminal acts can be suggested to the hypnotized subject which are just as certain to be performed by him as any other acts. Such a subject will discharge a blank-loaded pistol at any one, when told to do so, or stab him with a paper dagger. While admitting the facts, the Nancy theorists claim that the subject knows the performance to be a farce; gets suggestions of the unreality of it from the experimenters, and so acquiesces. This is probably true, as is seen in frequent cases in which patients have refused, in the hypnotic sleep, to perform suggested acts which shocked their modesty, veracity, etc. This goes to show that the Nancy school are right in saying that while, in hypnosis, suggestibility is exaggerated to an enormous degree, still it has limits in the more well-knit habits, moral sentiments, social opinions, etc., of the subjects. And it further shows that hypnosis is probably, as they claim, a temporary disturbance, rather than a pathological condition of mind and body.

There have been many remarkable and sensational cases of cure of disease by hypnotic suggestion reported, especially in France. That hysteria in all its manifold manifestations has been relieved is certainly true, but that any organic, structural disease has ever been cured by hypnotism is unproven. It is not regarded by medical authorities as an agent of much therapeutic value, and is rarely employed; but it is doubtful, in view of the natural prejudice caused by the pretensions of charlatans, whether its merits have been fairly tested.

Theory — Two rival theories are held as to the general character of hypnosis. The Paris school already referred to, led by Charcot, hold that it is a pathological condition which can be induced only in patients already mentally diseased, or having neuropathic tendencies. They claim that the three stages described above are a discovery of great importance. The so-called Nancy school, on the other hand, led by

Bernheim, deny the pathological character of hypnosis altogether, claiming that the hypnotic condition is nothing more than a special form of ordinary sleep brought on artificially by suggestion. Suggestion, they say, is only an exaggeration of an influence to which all persons are normally subject. All the variations, stages, curious phenomena, etc., of the Paris school, say they, can be explained by this 'suggestion' hypothesis. The Nancy school is completely victorious, as far as the great mass of the facts are concerned.

The facts show an intimacy of interaction between mind and body, to which current psychology in its psycho-physical theories is only beginning to do justice; and it is this aspect of the whole matter which I would emphasize in this connection. It will be observed that all the phases of 'suggestion' passed in review in earlier sections of this chapter get direct illustration from similar phenomena occurring in hypnosis. I need not cite them again in detail. The hypnotic condition of consciousness may, therefore, be taken to represent the thing called 'suggestion' most remarkably.

Law of Dynamogenesis

The facts of suggestion now given may be generalized under a so-called 'law,' which current psychology and biology agree in accepting as a well-established principle of the manifestations of organic and mental life. The principle of contractility recognized in biology simply states that all stimulations to living matter, — from protoplasm to the highest vegetable and animal structures, — if they take effect at all, tend to bring about movements or contractions in the mass of the organism. This is now also safely established as a phenomenon of consciousness — that every sensation or incoming process tends to bring about action or outgoing process. The facts of suggestion now set forth may be taken as, in so far, an array of evidence in support of what we may call, once for all, *Dynamogenesis*. Certain practical illustrations of it are given in the chapters which immediately precede: they show also the sure foundation of the method of studying children which I have based upon it. I shall accordingly expect no opposition to the use of this principle as the foundation-stone of the theory of organic development developed subsequently in this work' however faulty my presentation of it may be in the eyes of competent critics in either of these sciences.

In attempting, however, to reach some kind of formula of dynamogenesis we encounter a certain difficulty. For when we had occasion to inquire in an earlier place what the main character of all suggestion is, that character which constitutes its suggestion, we found definitions very conflicting; and gave as our own definition only the most general description of the reaction called suggestive, i.e. that it involved consciousness and issues in a movement more or less closely associated in earlier experience with the particular stimulus in question.

This, it is plain, constitutes suggestion a phenomenon of greater or less *habit*, taking hypnotic suggestion as type, in which prompt discharges in well-formed pathways is the striking fact. Numerous instances among the facts reported in this chapter come to mind. The statement ordinarily made in the more recent psychologies, to the effect that the idea of a movement is already the beginning of that movement, serves to generalize these facts, provided we understand by the 'idea of movement,' not merely the clear consciousness of a movement, but also the vaguest and most subconscious reminiscences, feelings, intimations of movement, which cluster or hang about or enter into, however meagrely, the state of mind which issues in the movement making up the suggested reaction.

But it is just as evident, when we recall the various

instances in detail, that they have another and different aspect. Very many suggestions seem to perform a function which is not exhausted when we say that they issue in movements. They issue in movements, it is true; but not in exactly the movements and those alone which have been associated with these stimuli before. Many of them seem to beget new movements, by a kind of adaptation of the organism — movements which are an evident improvement upon those which the organism has formerly accomplished.

To make this plain we have only to recall some cases from the reports made in this chapter and the earlier ones. The child reams handwriting by acting upon the suggestion which the copy set before him affords. How could he control his movements at all, if each suggestion called out only the movements which he had already learned? The child adapts himself again to persons, and differently to different persons, from week to week. How does he do this? Persons of course suggest action to him, but how does he manage to break up, in appropriate ways, the fixed organic tendencies to action in which we have found early bashfulness to consist? The child reams to estimate distance, and his visual experiences become, as we have seen, suggestions to him of hand movements remarkably adjusted to his reach and to the dimensions, etc., of things. How is this done? And so might more cases be cited.

This aspect of suggestion opens up what is one of the main problems of this book to discuss, the theory of *Accommodation*. It is only in point here to show that this thing, accommodation, is a fact, and that it consists in some influence in the organism which works directly in the face of habit. Suggestion works to break up habit.

We saw above, also, two views as to the presence and influence of consciousness in this matter of suggestion. Some theorists hold that there is no suggestion without consciousness; others that consciousness is not a necessary element. The dispute seems to turn upon the predominant recognition in reactions of one of the two tendencies, Habit or Accommodation. It is true and universal that consciousness tends to disappear from reactions as they are oftener repeated — as they become, that is, more habitual. The things we have reamed to do best, most definitely, most exactly, must *unalterably* in a word, these things require least thought, direction, feeling, consciousness. So with our reflex and semi-automatic actions: they come to go on, as pathological cases show, without the cortex of the brain, in cases when fainting or forgetfulness deprive us of all knowledge that we do them. On the other hand, we find that whenever there is accommodation — the breaking up of habit, the effort to learn, the acquirement of new movements, and co-ordinations of movement — there consciousness is present, and present in vivid and heightened form according as the habit fought against is fixed, and the road to the new acquisition an uphill road. The things most new, difficult, imperfect, hard to effect, these dwell in the very focus of our personal knowledge and attention.

[Rourtesy: J.M. Baldwin]

Select Bibliography

Abercrombie, M. L. J. (1960) *The Anatomy of Judgement: an Investigation into the Processes of Perception and Reasoning.* Hutchinson; reprinted Free Association Books, 1989.

Abram, K., & Teplin, L. (1991). Co-occurring disorders among mentally ill jail detainees: Implications for public policy. *American Psychologist, 46,* 1036–1046.

Adams, W., Kendell, R. E., Hare, E. H., & Munk-Jorgensen, P. (1993). Epidemiological evidence that maternal influenza contributes to the aetiology of schizophrenia. An analysis of Scottish, English, and Danish data. *British Journal of Psychiatry, 163,* 522–534.

Aguglia, E., Casacchia, M., Cassano, G. B., Faravelli, C., Ferrari, G., Giordano, P., Pancheri, P., Ravizza, L., Trabucchi, M., Bolino, F., Scarpato, A., Berardi, D., Provenzano, G., Brugnoli, R., & Rozzini, R. (1993). Double-blind study of the efficacy and safety of sertraline versus fluoxetine in major depression. *International Clinical Psychopharmacology, 8,* 197–202.

Aiken, L., Somers, S., & Shore, M. (1986). Private foundations in health affairs: A case study of a national initiative for the chronically mentally ill. *American Psychologist, 41,* 1290–1295.

Akbarian, S., Bunney, W. E. J., Potkin, S. G., Wigal, S. B., Hagman, J. O., Sandman, C. A., & Jones, E. G. (1993). Altered distribution of nicotinamide-adenine dinucleotide phosphate-diaphorase cells in frontal lobe of schizophrenics implies disturbances of cortical development. *Archives of General Psychiatry, 50,* 169–177.

Akiskal, H. S. (1985). Interaction of biologic and psychologic factors in the origin of depressive disorders. *Acta Psychiatrica Scandinavica., 319*(Suppl.), 131–139.

Alexander, M. J. (1996). Women with co-occurring addictive and mental disorders: An emerging profile of vulnerability. *American Journal of Orthopsychiatry, 66,* 61–70.

Alexander, P. C., Neimeyer, R. A., Follette, V. M., Moore, M. K., & Harter, S. (1989). A comparison of group treatments of women sexually abused as children. *Journal of Consulting and Clinical Psychology, 57,* 479–483.

Alexandris, Athina and Vaslamatzis, Grigoris, eds. (1993) *Countertransference: Theory, Technique, Teaching.* Karnac.

Allness, D. & Knoedler, W. (1999). *Recommended PACT standards for new teams* [On-line]. Available: http://www.nami.org/ about/pactstd.html

Alloy, L. B., & Abramson, L. Y. (1988). Depressive realism: Four theoretical perspectives. In Alloy L. B. (Ed.), *Cognitive processes in depression* (pp. 223–265). New York: Guilford Press.

Amacher, Peter (1965) *Freud's Neurological Education and Its Influence on Psychoanalytic Theory. Psychological Issues* Vol. 4 no. 4, Monograph 16. International Universities Press.

American Psychiatric Association (1994). *Diagnostic and statistical manual of mental disorders* (4th ed.). Washington, DC: Author.

American Psychiatric Association. (1993). *Practice guideline for major depressive disorder in adults. American Journal of Psychiatry, 150*(Suppl. 4), 1–26.

Andersson, C., Chakos, M., Mailman, R., & Lieberman, J. (1998). Emerging roles for novel antipsychotic medications in the treatment of schizophrenia. *Psychiatric Clinics of North America, 21,* 151–179.

Andrade, C., Gangadhar, B. N., Subbakrishna, D. K., Channabasavanna, S. M., & Pradhan, N. (1998). A double-blind comparision of sinusoidal wave and brief-pulse electroconvulsive therapy in endogenous depression. *Convulsive Therapy, 4,* 297–305.

Andreasen, N. C. (1995). Symptoms, signs, and diagnosis of schizophrenia. *Lancet, 346,* 477B-481.

Andreasen, N. C. (1997a). The evolving concept of schizophrenia: From Kraepelin to the present and future. *Schizophrenia Research, 28,* 105–109.

Andreasen, N. C. (1997b). Linking mind and brain in the study of mental illnesses: A project for a scientific psychopathology. *Science, 275,* 1586–1593.

Andreasen, N. C., O'Leary, D. S., Flaum, M., Nopoulos, P., Watkins, G. L., Boles Ponto, L. L., & Hichwa, R. D. (1997). Hypofrontality in schizophrenia: Distributed dysfunctional circuits in neuroleptic-naive patients. *Lancet, 349,* 1730–1734.

Andreasen, N. C., Paradiso, S., & O'Leary, D. S. (1998). "Cognitive dysmetria" as an integrative theory of schizophrenia: A dysfunction in cortical-subcortical-cerebellar circuitry? *Schizophrenia Bulletin, 24,* 203–218.

Angst, J., Angst, F., & Stassen, H. H. (1999). Suicide risk in patients with major depressive disorder. *Journal of Clinical Psychiatry, 60*(Suppl. 2), 57–62.

Anon. (1902) 'Phrenology', in *The New Volumes of the Encyclopedia Britannica, constituting... the Tenth Edition.* Edinburgh: Black, 1902, vol. 31, pp. 709-10.

Anzieu, Didier (1984) *The Group and the Unconscious.* Routledge & Kegan Paul.

Appleby, L., Desai, P. N., Luchins, D. J., Gibbons, R. D., & Hedeker, D. R. (1993). Length of stay and recidivism in schizophrenia: A study of public psychiatric hospital patients. *American Journal of Psychiatry, 150,* 72–76.

Arborelius, L., Owens, M. J., Plotsky, P. M., & Nemeroff, C. B. (1999). The role of corticotropin-releasing factor in depression and anxiety disorders. *Journal of Endocrinology, 160,* 1–12.

Arendt, Hannah (1963) *Eichmann in Jerusalem: A Report on the Banality of Evil.* N. Y.: Viking Penguin; revised and enlarged, 1965; reprinted Harmondsworth: Penguin, 1977.

Armitage, R., Rush, A. J., Trivedi, M., Cain, J., & Roffwarg, H. P. (1994). The effects of nefazodone on sleep architecture in depression. *Neuropsychopharmacology, 10,* 123–127.Arnold, S. E., Hyman, B. T., Van Hoesen, G. W., & Damasio, A. R. (1991). Some cytoarchitectural abnormalities of the entorhinal cortex in schizophrenia. *Archives of General Psychiatry, 48,* 625–632.

Ascher, J. A., Cole, J. O., Colin, J. N., Feighner, J. P., Ferris, R. M., Fibiger, H. C., Golden, R. N., Martin, P., Potter, W. Z., Richelson, E., & Sulser, F. (1995). Bupropion: A review of its mechanism of antidepressant activity. *Journal of Clinical Psychiatry, 56,* 395–401.

Atkinson, R. L. *et al.* (1990) *Introduction to Psychology,* 10th ed. Harcourt Brace Janovich.

Attkisson, C., Cook, J., Karno, M., Lehman, A., McGlashan, T. H., Meltzer, H. Y., O'Connor, M., Richardson, D., Rosenblatt, A., Wells, K., & Williams, J., & Hohmann, A. A. (1992). Clinical services research. *Schizophrenia Bulletin, 18,* 561–626.

Bach, Steven (1985) *Final Cut: Dreams and Disaster in the Making of Heaven's Gate.* Cape.

Bakan, David (1958) *Sigmund Freud and the Jewish Mystical Tradition;* reprinted Free Association Books, 1990.

Baldessarini, R. J., Cohen, B. M., & Teicher, M. H. (1990). Pharmacological treatment. In S. T. Levy & P. T Ninan (Eds.), *Schizophrenia: Treatment of acute psychotic episodes* (pp. 61–118). Washington, DC: American Psychiatric Press.

Baldwin, D. S., & Birtwistle, J. (1998). The side effect burden associated with drug treatment of panic disorder. *Journal of Clinical Psychiatry, 59*(Suppl. 8), 39–44.

Ballenger, J. C., Davidson, J. R., Lecrubier, Y., Nutt, D. J., Bobes, J., Beidel, D. C., Ono, Y., & Westenberg, H. G. (1998). Consensus statement on social anxiety disorder from the International Consensus Group on Depression and Anxiety. *Journal of Clinical Psychiatry, 59*(Suppl. 17), 54–60.

Ballus, C. (1997). Effects of antipsychotics on the clinical and psychosocial behavior of patients with schizophrenia. *Schizophrenia Research, 28*, 247–255.

Barbee, J. G. (1998). Mixed symptoms and syndromes of anxiety and depression: Diagnostic, prognostic, and etiologic issues. *Annals of Clinical Psychiatry, 10*, 15–29.

Barlow, D. H. (1988). *Anxiety and its disorders: The nature and treatment of anxiety and panic*, New York: Guilford Press.

Barlow, D. H., & Lehman, C. L. (1996). Advances in the psychosocial treatment of anxiety disorders. Implications for national health care. *Archives of General Psychiatry, 53*, 727–735.

Barlow, D. H., Chorpita, B. F., & Turovsky, J. (1996). Fear, panic, anxiety, and disorders of emotion. In D. A. Hope (Ed.), *Perspectives on anxiety, panic, and fear (The 43rd Annual Nebraska Symposium on Motivation*, pp. 251–328). Lincoln, NE: Nebraska University Press.

Barnes, T. R., & McPhillips, M. A. (1998). Novel antipsychotics, extrapyramidal side effects and tardive dyskinesia. *International Clinical Psychopharmacology, 13*(Suppl. 3), S49–S57.

Baron, M. (1997). Genetic linkage and bipolar affective disorder: Progress and pitfalls. *Molecular Psychiatry, 2*, 200–210.

Barta, P. E., Pearlson, G. D., Powers, R. E., Richards, S. S., & Tune, L. E. (1990). Auditory hallucinations and smaller superior temporal gyral volume in schizophrenia. *American Journal of Psychiatry, 147,* 1457–1462.

Basso, M. R., Nasrallah, H. A., Olson, S. C., & Bornstein, R. A. (1997). Cognitive deficits distinguish patients with adolescent- and adult-onset schizophrenia. *Neuropsychiatry, Neuropsychology, and Behavioral Neurology, 10,* 107–112.

Basso, M. R., Nasrallah, H. A., Olson, S. C., & Bornstein, R. A. (1998). Neuropsychological correlates of negative, disorganized and psychotic symptoms in schizophrenia. *Schizophrenia Research, 31,* 99–111.

Bauer, M. S., Calabrese, J., Dunner, D. L., Post, R., Whybrow, P. C., Gyulai, L., Tay, L. K., Younkin, S. R., Bynum, D., Lavori, P., & Price, R. A. (1994). Multisite data reanalysis of the validity of rapid cycling as a course modifier for bipolar disorder in DSM-IV. *American Journal of Psychiatry, 151,* 506–515.

Baxter, L. R., Jr., Mazziotta, J. C., Phelps, M. E., Selin, C. E., Guze, B. H., & Fairbanks, L. (1987). Cerebral glucose metabolic rates in normal human females versus normal males. *Psychiatry Research, 21,* 237–245.

Beasley, C. M., Jr., Dornseif, B. E., Bosomworth, J. C., Sayler, M. E., Rampey, A. H., Jr., Heiligenstein, J. H., Thompson, V. L., Murphy, D. J., & Masica, D. N. (1991). Fluoxetine and suicide: A meta-analysis of controlled trials of treatment for depression. *British Medical Journal, 303,* 685–692.

Beasley, C. M., Jr., Sayler, M. E., Cunningham, G. E., Weiss, A. M., & Masica, D. N. (1990). Fluoxetine in tricyclic refractory major depressive disorder. *Journal of Affective Disorders, 20,* 193–200.

Bebbington, P., & Kuipers, L. (1994). The predictive utility of expressed emotion in schizophrenia: An aggregate analysis. *Psychological Medicine, 24,* 707–718.

Beck, A. T. (1976). *Cognitive therapy and the emotional disorders.* New York: International Universities Press.

Beck, A. T., Rush A. J., & Shaw B. F. (1979). *Cognitive therapy of depression.* New York: Guilford Press.

Bell, C. C. & Mehta, H. (1981). The misdiagnosis of black patients with manic depressive illness. *Journal of the National Medical Association 73,* 101–107.

Bell, David. (1992) 'Hysteria — A Contemporary Kleinian Perspective', *Brit. J. Psychother.* 9: 169-80.

Bell, M. D., & Lysaker, P. H. (1997). Clinical benefits of paid work activity in schizophrenia: 1-year followup. *Schizophrenia Bulletin, 23,* 317–328.

Bell, M. D., & Ryan, E. R. (1984). Integrating psychosocial rehabilitation into the hospital psychiatric service. *Hospital and Community Psychiatry, 35,* 1017–1022.

Bell, M. D., Lysaker, P. H., & Milstein, R. M. (1996). Clinical benefits of paid work activity in schizophrenia. *Schizophrenia Bulletin, 22,* 51–67.

Bellack, A. S., & Mueser, K. T. (1993). Psychosocial treatment for schizophrenia. *Schizophrenia Bulletin, 19,* 317–336.

Berke, Joseph (1989) *The Tyranny of Malice: Exploring the Dark Side of Character and Culture.* Simon and Schuster.

Berkhofer, Robert. F. Jr. (1978) *The White Man's Indian: Images of the American Indian from Columbus to the Present.* N. Y.: Knopf; reprinted N. Y.: Vintage Books, 1979.

Bernal, Martin (1987) *Black Athena: The Afroasiatic Roots of Classical Civilisation. Vol. 1: The Fabrication of Ancient Greece 1785-1985.* Free Association Books.

Bernfeld, Siegfried (1944) 'Freud's Earliest Theories and the School of Helmholtz', *Psychonal. Quart.* 13: 341-62.

Berren, M., Hill, K., Merikle, E., Gonzalez, N., & Santiago, J. (1994). Serious mental illness and mortality rates. *Hospital and Community Psychiatry, 45,* 604–605.

Berry, David (1983) 'Science in Society', *New Statesman* 28 Oct., pp. 10-12.

Bertelsen, A., Harvald, B., & Hauge, M. (1977). A Danish twin study of manic-depressive disorders. *British Journal of Psychiatry, 130,* 330–351.

Besio, S. W., & Mahler, J. (1993). Benefits and challenges of using consumer staff in supported housing services. *Hospital and Community Psychiatry, 44,* 490–491.

Bettleheim, Bruno (1983) *Freud and Man's Soul.* Chatto and Windus/Hogarth.

Bezold, H. S., MacDowell M., & Kunkel R. (1996). Predicting psychiatric length of stay. *Administration and Policy in Mental Health, 23,* 407–423.

Bierut, L. J., Heath, A. C., Bucholz, K. K., Dinwiddie, S. H., Madden, P. A., Statham, D. J., Dunne, M. P., & Martin, N. G. (1999). Major depressive disorder in a community-based twin sample: Are there different genetic and environmental contributions for men and women? *Archives of General Psychiatry, 56,* 557–563.

Bion, Wilfred R. (1955) 'Group Dynamics — a Re-view', in Klein *et al.*, eds. (1955), pp. 440-77; reprinted in Bion (1961), pp. 141-91.

Black, D. W., Winokur, G., & Nasrallah, A. (1987). The treatment of depression: Electroconvulsive therapy v antidepressants: A naturalistic evaluation of 1,495 patients. *Comprehensive Psychiatry, 28,* 169–182.

Blackburn, I. M., Eunson, K. M., & Bishop, S. (1986). A two-year naturalistic follow-up of depressed patients treated with cognitive therapy, pharmacotherapy and a combination of both. *Journal of Affective Disorders, 10,* 67–75.

Blanchard, J. J., Mueser, K. T., & Bellack, A. S. (1998). Anhedonia, positive and negative affect, and social functioning in schizophrenia. *Schizophrenia Bulletin, 24,* 413–424.

Blehar, M. C., DePaulo, J. R. Jr, Gershon, E. S., Reich, T., Simpson, S. G., & Nurnberger, J. I. Jr. (1998). Women with bipolar disorder: Findings from the NIMH Genetics Initiative sample. *Psychopharmacology Bulletin, 34,* 239–243.

Blejer, J. (1966) 'Psychoanalysis of the Psycho-analytic Frame', *Int. J. Psycho-Anal.* 48: 511-19.

Bloor, David (1976) *Knowledge and Social Imagery.* Routledge & Kegan Paul.

Blumenthal, S. J. (1988). Suicide: A guide to risk factors, assessment, and treatment of suicidal patients. *Medical Clinics of North America, 72,* 937–971.

Blumenthal, S. J. (1994a). Gender differences in mental disorders. *Journal of Clinical Psychiatry, 3,* 453–458.

Blumenthal, S. J. (1994b). Women and depression. *Journal of Women's Health, 3,* 467–453.

Bogerts, B., Lieberman, J. A., Ashtari, M., Bilder, R. M., Degreet, G., & Lerner, G. (1993). Hippocampus-amygdala volumes and psychopathology in chronic schizophrenia. *Biological Psychiatry, 33,* 236–246.

Bolden-Watson, C., & Richelson, E. (1993). Blockade by newly-developed antidepressants of biogenic amine uptake into rat brain synaptosomes. *Life Sciences, 52,* 1023–1029.

Bollas, Christopher (1987) 'Expressive Uses of the Counter-transference', in *The Shadow of the Object: Psychoanalysis of the Unthought Known.* Free Association Books, pp. 200-35.

Bond, G. R., & Dincin, J. (1986). Accelerating entry into transitional employment in a psychosocial rehabilitation agency. *Rehabilitation Psychology, 31,* 143–154.

Bond, G. R., Drake, R. E., Mueser, K. T., & Becker, D. R. (1997). An update on supported employment for people with severe mental illness. *Psychiatric Services, 48,* 335–346.

Bond, G. R., McGrew, J. H., & Fekete, D. M. (1995). Assertive outreach of frequent users of psychiatric hospitals: A meta-analysis. *Journal of Mental Health Administration, 22*, 4–16.

Boorman, John (1985) *Money into Light: The Emerald Forest. A Diary*. Faber and Faber.

Borkman, T. J. (1991). Self-help groups. Introduction to the special issue. *American Journal of Community Psychology, 19*, 643–650.

Borland, A., McRae, J., & Lycan, C. (1989). Outcome of five years of continuous intensive case management. *Hospital and Community Psychiatry, 40*, 369–376.

Bowden, C. L., Brugger, A. M., Swann, A. C., Calabrese, J. R., Janicak, P. G., Petty, F., Dilsaver, S. C., Davis, J. M., Rush, A. J., Small, J. G., Garza-Treviño, E. S., Risch, S. C., Goodnick, P. J., & Morris, D. D. (1994). Efficacy of divalproex vs lithium and placebo in the treatment of mania. The Depakote Mania Study Group. *Journal of the American Medical Association, 271*, 918–924.

Bower, Tom (1991) *Maxwell: The Outsider*. William Heinemann.

Bracha, H. S. (1991). Etiology of structural asymmetry in schizophrenia: An alternative hypothesis. *Schizophrenia Bulletin, 17*, 551–553.

Brady, Frank (1990) *Citizen Welles: A Biography of Orson Welles*. Hodder and Stoughton.

Branden, Barbara (1986) *The Passion of Ayn Rand: A Biography*. N. Y.: Doubleday.

Braun, C. M., Lapierre, D., Hodgins, S., Toupin, J., Leveille, S., & Constantineau, C. (1995). Neurological soft signs in schizophrenia: Are they related to negative or positive symptoms, neuropsychological performance and violence? *Archives of Clinical Neuropsychology, 10*, 489–509.

Brazo, P., & Dollfus, S. (1997). Syndromic and diagnostic heterogeneity of schizophrenia. *Encephale, 23,* 20–24.

Breggin, P. R., & Breggin, G. R. (1994). *Talking back to Prozac.* New York: St. Martin's Press.

Breiter, H. C., Etcoff, N. L., Whalen, P. J., Kennedy, W. A., Rauch, S. L., Buckner, R. L., Strauss, M. M., Hyman, S. E., & Rosen, B. R. (1996). Response and habituation of the human amygdala during visual processing of facial expression. *Neuron, 17,* 875–887.

Brekke, J. S., & Barrio, C. (1997). Cross-ethnic symptom differences in schizophrenia: The influence of culture and minority status. *Schizophrenia Bulletin, 23,* 305–316.

Brekke, J. S., Raine, A., & Thomson, C. (1995). Cognitive and psychophysiological correlates of positive, negative, and disorganized symptoms in the schizophrenia spectrum. *Psychiatry Research, 57,* 241–250.

Brenman Pick, I. (1985) 'Working Through in the Counter-transference', *Int. J. Psycho-anal.* 66: 157-66; reprinted in Spillius, ed. (1988), vol. 2, pp. 34-47.

Breslau, N., Davis, G. C., Andreski, P., & Peterson, E. (1991). Traumatic events and posttraumatic stress disorder in an urban population of young adults. *Archives of General Psychiatry, 48,* 216–222.

Breslau, N., Kessler, R. C., Chilcoat, H. D., Schultz, L. R., Davis, G. C., & Andreski, P. (1998). Trauma and posttraumatic stress disorder in the community: The 1996 Detroit Area Survey of Trauma. *Archives of General Psychiatry, 55,* 626–632.

Breuer, Josef and Freud, Sigmund (1895) *Studies on Hysteria.,* in Freud (1953-73), vol. 2.

Britton, Ronald (1989) 'The Missing Link: Parental Sexuality in the Oedipus Complex', in Britton *et al.* (1989), pp. 83-102.

Brixey, S. N., Gallagher, B. J., III, McFalls, J. A., Jr., & Parmelee, L. F. (1993). Gestational and neonatal factors in the etiology of schizophrenia. *Journal of Clinical Psychology, 49*, 447–456.

Broadhead, W. E., Blazer, D. G., George, L. K., & Tse, C. K. (1990). Depression, disability days, and days lost from work in a prospective epidemiologic survey. *Journal of the American Medical Association, 264*, 2524–2528.

Brody, S. (1980) 'Transitional Objects: Idealisation of a Phenomenon', *Psychoanal. Quart.* 49: 561-605.

Brown, Dee (1978) *Bury My Heart at Wounded Knee: An Indian History of the American West.* Chatto.

Brown, G. W., & Harris, T. O. (1989). *Life events and illness.* New York: Guilford Press.

Brown, G. W., & Moran, P. M. (1997). Single mothers, poverty and depression. *Psychological Medicine, 27*, 21–33.

Brown, G. W., Harris, T. O., & Hepworth, C. (1994). Life events and endogenous depression. A puzzle reexamined. *Archives of General Psychiatry, 51*, 525–534.

Brown, S. (1997). Excess mortality of schizophrenia—A meta-analysis. *British Journal of Psychiatry, 171*, 502–508.

Browne, A., & Finkelhor, D. (1986). Impact of child sexual abuse: A review of the research. *Psychological Bulletin, 99*, 66–77.

Bruner, Jerome (1951) 'Personality Dynamics and the Process of Perceiving', in R. V. Blake and G. V. Ramsey, eds. *Perception: an Approach to Personality.* New York: Ronald Press.

Buchanan, R. W. (1995). Clozapine: Efficacy and safety. *Schizophrenia Bulletin, 21*, 579–591.

Buchanan, R. W., Breier, A., Kirkpatrick, B., Elkashef, A., Munson, R. C., Gellad, F., Carpenter, W. T., Jr. (1993). Structural abnormalities in deficit and non-deficit schizophrenia. *American Journal of Psychiatry, 150,* 59–65.

Buckley, P. F. (1997). New dimensions in the pharmacologic treatment of schizophrenia and related psychoses. *Journal of Clinical Pharmacology, 37,*' 363–378.

Buckser, Andrew S. (1992) 'Lynching as Ritual in the American South', *Berkeley J. Sociol.* 37:11-28.

Burke, K. C., Burke, J. D., Jr., Regier, D. A., & Rae, D. S. (1990). Age at the onset of selected mental disorders in five community populations. *Archives of General Psychiatry, 47,* 511–518.

Burke, M. J., Silkey, B., & Preskorn, S. H. (1994). Pharmacoeconomic considerations when evaluating treatment options for major depressive disorder. *Journal of Clinical Psychiatry, 55*(Suppl. A), 42–52.

Burtt, Edwin. A. (1932) *The Metaphysical Foundations of Modern Physical Science*, 2nd ed., Routledge.

Buscombe, Ed (1988) *The BFI Companion to the Western.* Deutsch.

Bymaster, F. P., Rasmussen, K., Calligaro, D. O., Nelson, D. L., DeLapp, N. W., Wong, D. T., & Moore, N. A. (1997). In vitro and in vivo biochemistry of olanzapine: A novel, atypical antipsychotic drug. *Journal of Clinical Psychiatry, 58*(Suppl. 10), 28–36.

Cadenhead, K. S., Geyer, M. A., Butler, R. W., Perry, W., Sprock, J., & Braff, D. L. (1997). Information processing deficits of schizophrenia patients: Relationship to clinical ratings, gender and medication status. *Schizophrenia Research, 28,* 51–62.

Calabrese, J. R., & Delucchi, G. A. (1990). Spectrum of efficacy of valproate in 55 patients with rapid-cycling bipolar disorder. *American Journal of Psychiatry, 147,* 431–434.

Callahan, D. (1999). Balancing efficiency and need in allocating resources to the care of persons with serious mental illness. *Psychiatric Services, 50,* 664–666.

Callahan, E. J., Bertakis, K. D., Azari, R., Robbins, J., Helms, L. J., & Miller, J. (1996). The influence of depression on physician-patient interaction in primary care. *Family Medicine, 28,* 346–351.

Camus, Albert (1955) 'The Myth of Sisyphus' in *The Myth of Sisyphus and Other Essays.* N.Y.: Knopf; reprinted N. Y.: Vintage, pp. 88-91.

Cannon, Lou (1991) *President Reagan: The Role of a Lifetime.* Simon and Schuster.

Cannon, T. D., Kaprio, J., Lonnqvist, J., Huttunen, M., & Koskenvuo, M. (1998). The genetic epidemiology of schizophrenia in a Finnish twin cohort. A population-based modeling study. *Archives of General Psychiatry, 55,* 67–74.

Capleton, R. A. (1996). Cognitive function in schizophrenia: Association with negative and positive symptoms. *Psychological Reports, 78,* 123–128.

Cardno, A. G., & Farmer, A. E. (1995). The case for or against heterogeneity in the etiology of schizophrenia. The genetic evidence. *Schizophrenia Research, 17,* 153–159.

Carew, Jan (1988) 'Columbus and the Origins of Racism in the Americas', *Race and Class* 29:1-19; 30:33-57.

Carling, P. (1989). Access to housing: Cornerstone of the American dream. *Journal of Rehabilitation, 55,* 6–8.

Casey, D. E. (1997). The relationship of pharmacology to side effects. *Journal of Clinical Psychiatry, 58*(Suppl. 10), 55–62.

Cassens, G., Inglis, A. K., Appelbaum, P. S., & Gutheil, T. G. (1990). Neuroleptics: Effects on neuropsychological function in chronic schizophrenic patients. *Schizophrenia Bulletin, 16,* 477–499.

Cassirer, Ernst (1953-57) *The Philosophy of Symbolic Forms,* 3 vols. Yale University Press.

Castrogiovanni, P., Iapichino, S., Pacchierotti, C., & Pieraccini, F. (1998). Season of birth in psychiatry. A review. *Neuropsychobiology, 37,* 175–181.

Cazzullo, C. L., Bertrando, P., Clerici, C., Bressi, C., Da Ponte, C., & Albertini, E. (1989). The efficacy of an information group intervention on relatives of schizophrenics. *International Journal of Social Psychiatry, 35,* 313–323.

Center for Mental Health Services. (1995). *Double jeopardy: Persons with mental illnesses in the criminal justice system.* Rockville, MD: Author.

Center for Mental Health Services. (1997). *Cultural competence standards in managed mental health care for four underserved/ underrepresented racial/ethnic groups* (Final report from Working Groups on Cultural Competence in Managed Mental Health Care). Rockville, MD: Author.

Center for Mental Health Services. (1998). *Electroconvulsive therapy background paper* (DHHS Publication No. SMA 98-3201). Vienna, VA: Research-Abele, Inc.

Chakos, M. H., Alvir, J. M., Woerner, M. G., Koreen, A., Geisler, S., Mayerhoff, D., Sobel, S., Kane, J. M., Borenstein, M., & Lieberman, J. A. (1996). Incidence and correlates of tardive dyskinesia in first episode of schizophrenia. *Archives of General Psychiatry, 53,* 313–319.

Chamberlin, J., & Rogers, J. A. (1990). Planning a community-based mental health system. Perspective of service recipients. *American Psychologist, 45,* 1241–1244.

Chambless, D. K., Baker, M. J., Baucom, D. H., Beutler, L. E., et al. (1998). Update on empirically validated therapies II. *The Clinical Psychologist, 51,* 3–16.

Charney, D. S., & Deutch, A. (1996). A functional neuroanatomy of anxiety and fear: Implications for the pathophysiology and treatment of anxiety disorders. *Critical Reviews in Neurobiology, 10,* 419–446.

Chouinard, G. (1988). The use of benzodiazepines in the treatment of manic-depressive illness. *Journal of Clinical Psychiatry, 49*(Suppl.), 15–20.

Christensen, A., & Heavey, C. L. (1999). Interventions for couples. *Annual Review of Psychology, 50,* 165B-190.

Ciompi, L. (1980). Catamnestic long-term study on the course of life and aging of schizophrenics. *Schizophrenia Bulletin, 6,* 606–618.

Claghorn, J. L., & Feighner, J. P. (1993). A double-blind comparison of paroxetine with imipramine in the long-term treatment of depression. *Journal of Clinical Psychopharmacology, 13,* 23S–27S.

Clark, L. A., Watson, D., & Mineka, S. (1994). Temperament, personality, and the mood and anxiety disorders. *Journal of Abnormal Psychology, 103,* 103–116.

Clayton, P. J., & Darvish, H. S. (1979). Course of depressive symptoms following the stress of bereavement. In J. E. Barrett, R. M. Rose, & G. Klerman (Eds.), *Stress and mental disorder* (pp. 121–136). New York: Raven.

Cocks, G. and Crosby, T. L. (1987) *Psychohistory: Readings in the Method of Psychology, Psychoanalysis, and History.* Yale.

Cohen, C. I. (1993). Poverty and the course of schizophrenia: Implications for research and policy. *Hospital and Community Psychiatry, 44,* 951–958.

Colman, A, D. and Bexton, W. H. (1975) *Group Relations Reader 1.* Washington, D. C.: A. K. Rice Institute.

Coltart, Nina (1986a) '"Slouching toward s Bethlehem"...or Thinking the Unthinkable in Psychoanalysis', in Kohon (1986), pp. 185-99.; reprinted in *Slouching towards Bethlehem... and Further Psychoanalytic Explorations.* Free Association Books, 1992, pp. 1-14.

Cooper, David (1972) *The Death of the Family.* Harmondsworth: Penguin.

Creme, Phyllis (1991) 'Winnicott and the Cinema', paper read to annual conference of THERIP (The Higher Education Network for Research and Teaching in Psychoanalysis).

Darwin, Charles R. (1874) *The Descent of Man, and Selection in Relation to Sex*, 2nd ed., revised and augmented. Murray, 1889.

Davidson, Basil (1987) 'The Ancient World and Africa: Whose Roots? *Race & Class* 29: 1-15,1987.

Davis, Madeleine and Wallbridge, David (1981) *Boundary and Space: An Introduction the Work of D. W. Winnicott.* Karnac; reprinted Harmondsworth: Penguin, 1983.

Descartes, René (1637) *Discourse on the Method of Properly Conducting One's Reason and of Seeking the Truth in the Sciences*, in *Discourse on Method and The Meditations.* Harmondsworth: Penguin, 1968, pp. 25-91.

Deutsch, Felix, ed. (1959) *On the Mysterious Leap from the Mind to the Body: A Workshop Study of the Theory of Conversion.* N. Y.: International Universities Press.

Dollard, John (1937) *Caste and Class in a Southern Town.* reprinted Garden City, N. Y.: Doubleday Anchor, 1957.

Dunne, J. G. (1982) 'Chinatowns', *New York Review of Books.* 21 October, pp. 6-10.

During, Simon, ed. (1993)*The Cultural Studies Reader.* Routledge.

Dworkin, Dennis L. and Roman, Leslie G. (1993) *Views Beyond the Border Country: Raymond Williams and Cultural Politics.* Routledge.

Epstein, L. and Feiner, A. H. (1983) *Countertransference: The Therapist's Contribution to the Therapeutic Situation.* Aronson.

Faimberg, Haydée (1988) 'The Telescoping of Generations: Genealogy of Certain Identifications', *Contemp. Psychoanal.* 24: 99-118.

Fairbairn, W. Ronald D. (1952) *Psychoanalytic Studies of the Personality.* Routledge & Kegan Paul.

Feldman, Michael (1992) 'Splitting and Projective identification', in Anderson, ed. (1992), pp. 74-88.

Fenichel, Otto (1941) *Problems in Psychoanalytic Technique,* New York: Psychoanalytic Quarterly.

Figlio, Karl (1978) 'Chlorosis and Chronic Disease in Nineteenth-century Britain: the Social Constitution of Somatic Illness in a Capitalist Society', *Internat. J. Health Services* 8: 589-617.

Finlay, Marike (1989) 'Post-Modernizing Psychoanalysis/ Psychoanalysing Post-Modernity', *Free Assns.* 16: 43-80.

Foucault, Michel (1967) *Madness and Civilisation: A History of Insanity in the Age of Reason.* Tavistock.

Foulkes, S. H. (1948) *Introduction to Group-Analytic Psychotherapy.* Heinemann Medical; reprinted Maresfield, 1983.

Freeman, Jo (1970) 'The Tyranny of Structurelessness', pamphlet reprinted in *Berkeley J. Sociol.*; reprinted Leeds Women, n.d.

Freud, Sigmund (1891) *On Aphasia: A Critical Study.* N. Y.: International Universities Press, 1953.

Fromm, Erich (1941) *Fear of Freedom;* U. S. title - *Escape from Freedom.* N. Y.: Rinehart & Co.

Frosh, Stephen (1991) *Identity Crisis: Modernity, Psychoanalysis and the Self.* Macmillan

Gay, Peter (1988) *Freud: A Life for Our Time.* Dent.

Gedo, John. E. (1986) *Conceptual Issues in Psychoanalysis: Essays in History and Method.* New York: Analytic Press.

Giovacchini, P. L. (1989) *Countertransference: Triumphs and Catastrophes.* Aronson.

Glover, Edward (1927) 'Lectures on Technique in Psychoanalysis', *Int. J. Psycho-Anal.* 8: 311-38.

Goffman, Erving (1961) *Asylums.* N. Y.: Anchor Books.

Green, André (1978) 'Potential Space in Psychoanalysis: The Object in the Setting', in Grolnick *et al.*, eds. (1978), pp. 167-90.

Greenberg, Jay R. and Mitchell, Stephen A. (1983) *Object Relations in Psychoanalytic Theory.* Harvard.

Grinberg, L. (1990) *The Goals of Psychoanalysis: Identification, Identity and Supervision.* Karnac.

Grolnick, S. *et al.*, eds. (1978) *Between Reality and Fantasy Transitional Objects and Phenomena.* Aronson.

Grossberg, Larry *et al.*, eds. (1992) *Cultural Studies.* Routledge.

Grosskurth, Phyllis (1986) *Melanie Klein: Her World and Her Work.* Hodder and Stoughton.

Grotstein, James (1981) *Splitting and Projective Identification.* Aronson.

Hann-Kende, F. (1933) 'On the role of Transference and Countertransference in Psychoanalysis', in Devereux, ed. (1953).

Haraway, Donna (1989) *Primate Visions: Gender, Race, and Nature in the World of Modern Science.* Routledge.

Harris, Emmylou and Nelson, Willie (1990) 'Gulf Coast Highway', Emmylou Harris, *Duets.* Reprise 7599-25791-2.

Hartmann, Heinz (1958) *Ego Psychology and the Problem of Adaptation.* N. Y.: International Universities Press.

Hinshelwood, Robert D. (1987) *What Happens in Groups.* Free Association Books.

Hodges, Andrew (1983) *Alan Turing: The Enigma of Intelligence.* Burnett Books/Hutchinson; reprinted Unwin Counterpoint, 1985.

Holland, Sue. and Holland, Ray (1984) 'Depressed Women: Outposts of Empire and Castles of Skin', in B. Richards, ed. (1984), pp. 92-101.

Horowitz, L. (1983) 'Projective Identification in Dyads and Groups', *Int. J. Group. Psychother.* 33: 259-79. reprinted in Colman and Geller, eds. (1985), pp. 21-35.

Horton, Robin (1967) 'African Traditional Thought and Western Science' *Africa* 37: 50-71, 155-87.

Huxley, Thomas. H. (1865) 'Emancipation — Black and White', in *Lay Sermons, Addresses and Reviews*. Macmillan, 1903, pp. 17-23.

Ingleby, David (1972) 'Ideology and the Human Sciences: Some Comments on the Role of Reification in Psychology and Psychiatry', in T. Pateman, ed., *Counter Course: A Handbook for Course Criticism*. Harmondsworth: Penguin, pp. 51-81.

Isaacs, Susan (1952) 'The Nature and Function of Phantasy', in Klein *et al.* (1952), pp. 67-121.

Jacoby, Russell (1981) *Dialectic of Defeat: Contours of Western Marxism*. Cambridge.

Jaques, Elliott (1951) *The Changing Culture of a Factory: A Study of Authority and Participation in an Industrial Setting*. Routledge & Kegan Paul.

Jay, Martin (1973) *The Dialectical Imagination: A History of the Frankfurt School and the Institute of Social Research, 1923-1950*. Little, Brown & Co.

Jones, Ernest (1949) *Hamlet and Oedipus*. N. Y.: Doubleday Anchor.

Kahne, M. J. (1967) 'On the Persistence of Transitional Phenomena into Adult Life', *Int. J. Psycho-Anal*, 48: 247-58.

Kahrl, W. L. (1982)*Water and Power: The Conflict over Los Angeles' Water Supply in the Owens Valley*. University of California Press.

Kaufman, M. Ralph and Heiman, Marcel, eds. (1964) *Evolution of Psychosomatic Concepts. Anorexia Nervosa: A Paradigm. N. Y.: International Universities Press.*

Keller, Helen (1903) *The Story of My Life.*; reprinted N. Y.: Scholastic Book Services, 1967.

Kelly, Kitty (1986) *His Way: The Unauthorised Biography of Frank Sinatra.* N. Y.: Bantam.

King, Pearl. & Steiner, Ricardo, eds. (1991) *The Freud-Klein Controversies 1941-45.* Tavistock/Routledge.

Klein, Melanie (1928) 'Early Stages of the Oedipus Conflict', reprinted in *W. M. K.* I, pp. 186-98.

Klein, Sydney (1980) 'Autistic Phenomena in Neurotic Patients', *Internat. J. Psycho-Anal.* 61:395-402.

Koenigsberg, R. A. (1977) *The Psychoanalysis of Racism, Revolution and Nationalism.* N. Y.: Library of Social Science.

Kogan, Ilony (1989) 'The Search for the Self', *Int. J. Psycho-Anal.* 70: 661-71.

Kohon, Gregorio (1985) 'Objects are Not People', *Free Assns.* 2: 19-30.

Kovel, Joel (1970) *White Racism: A Psychohistory.* N. Y. Pantheon; reprinted Free Association Books, 1988.

Kreeger, Lionel, ed. (1975) *The Large Group: Dynamics and Therapy.* Constable; reprinted Maresfield.

Kren, George (1987) 'The Holocaust and the Foundations of Moral Judgement', *J. Value Inquiry* 21: 55-64.

Kris, Ernst (1950) 'The Significance of Freud's Earliest Discoveries', *Int. J. Psycho-Anal.* 31: 108-16.

Kuhlenbeck, Hertwig (1957) *Brain and Consciousness: Some Prolegomena to an Approach of the Problem.* Basel/N. Y.: Karger.

Laing, Ronald D. (1960) *The Divided Self.: An Existential Study in Sanity and Madness.* Tavistock; reprinted Penguin, 1965.

Langer, Suzanne K. (1942) *Philosophy in a New Key: A Study in the Symbolism of Reason, Rite and Art.* Cambridge, MA: Harvard University Press.

Langs, Robert and Searles, Harold F. (1980) *Intrapsychic and Interpersonal Dimensions of Treatment: A Clinical Dialogue.* Aronson.

Laplanche, Jean and Pontalis, J.-B. (1983) *The Language of Psycho-Analysis.* Hogarth; reprinted Maresfield.

Las Casas, Bartolomé de (1552) *The Devastation of the Indes: A Brief Account.* Johns Hopkins, 1992.

Lash, Joseph. P. (1971) *Eleanor and Franklin: The Story of Their Relationship, based on Eleanor Roosevelt's Papers.* N. Y.: Norton.

Lasswell, Harold. D. (1930) *Psychopathology and Politics.* N. Y.: Viking.

Lerner, Leila, ed. (1992) *Illusion and Culture: A Tribute to Winnicott,* special issue of *Psychoanal. Rev.* 79 (no. 2).

Levidow, Les (1978) 'A Marxist critique of the IQ debate', *Radical Sci. J.* 6/7: 13-72.

Lorenz, Konrad (1961) *King Solomon's Ring.* Methuen.

Low, Barbara (1935) 'The psychological Compensation of the Analyst'. *Int. J. Psycho-Anal.* 16: 1-8.

Lowenberg, Peter (1985) *Decoding the Past: The Psychohistorical Approach.* University of California Press.

Lowenstein, R. M. (1963) 'Some Considerations on Free Association', J. *Amer. Psychoanal. Assn.* 11:451-73.

Lynn, Kenneth S. (1987) *Hemmingway.* Simon and Schuster.

McBride, Joseph (1992) *Frank Capra: The Catastrophe of Success.* Faber and Faber.

McDougall, Joyce (1980) 'Countertransference and Primitive Communication', in *Plea for a Measure of Abnormality.* Madison, CT: International Universities Press; reprinted Free Association Books, 1990, pp. 247-98.

Meltzer, D. and Harris Williams, M. (1988) *The Apprehension of Beauty: The Role of Aesthetic Conflict in Development, Art and Violence.* Strath Tay: Clunie Press.

Menninger, Karl (1938) *Man Against Himself.* Rupert Hart Davis; reprinted Harvest/HBJ.

Miller, Eric (1990) 'Experiential Learning Groups I: The Development of the Leicester Model', in E. Trist and H, Murray, eds., *The Social Engagement of Social Science: A Tavistock Anthology, Vol. 1: The Socio-Psychological Perspective.* Free Association Books, pp. 165-85.

Myrdal, Gunnar *et al.* (1944) *An American Dilemma: The Negro Problem and Modern Democracy.* N.Y.: Harper. N. Y.: Holt, Rinehart & Winston.

Nelson, Willie (1981) 'I'd Have to be Crazy', *Willie Nelson's Greatest Hits (and Some that Will Be).* Columbia CGK 37542.

O'Shea, James (1991) *The Daisy Chain: How Borrowed Billions Sank a Texas S&L.* Simon and Schuster.

Ogden, Thomas K. (1979) 'On Projective Identification', *Int. J. Psycho-Anal.* 60: 357-73.

Orr, D. W. (1988) 'Transference and Countertransference: a Historical Survey', in Wolstein, ed. (1988), pp. 91-110.

Perry, G. (1991) 'The First Face of America', *Sunday Times Magazine Section,* 3 Feb., pp. 19-24.

Racker, Heinrich (1968) *Transference and Countertransference.* Hogarth; reprinted Maresfield Reprints, 1982.

Rafaelsen, Lise (1992) 'Glimpses of Projective Identification in Inpatient Groups and in Life', *Group Anal.* 25: 55-59.

Rank, Otto (1912) *The Incest Theme in Literature and Legend: Fundamentals of a Psychology of Literary Creation.* Johns Hopkins University Press, 1992.

Rapaport, David (1959) 'The Structure of Psychoanalytic Theory: a Systematizing Attempt', in S. Koch, ed., *Psychology: A Study of a Science. Study I: Conceptual and Systematic.* Vol. 3: *Formulations of the Person in the Social Context.* N. Y.: McGraw-Hill, pp. 55-183; reprinted *Psychological Issues,* Vol. 2 no. 2, Monograph 6, 1960.

Rayner, Eric (1991) *The Independent Mind in British Psychoanalysis*. Free Association Books.

Rayner, Jay (1993) 'Ghetto v. Ghetto', *The Guardian Weekend*, 17 April 1993, pp. 22-34.

Reich, Annie (1951) 'On Countertransference'. *Int. J. Psycho-Anal.* 32: 25-31.

Reich, Wilhelm (1933) *Character Analysis: Principles and Techniques for Psychoanalysts in Practice and Training*, 2nd ed., New York: Orgone Institute.

Rex, John and Mason, David, eds. (1986) *Theories of Race and Ethnic Relations*. Cambridge. University Press.

Rieff, Philip (1960) *Freud: The Mind of the Moralist*. Gollancz, 3rd ed., Chicago, 1979.

Rorty, Richard (1980) *Philosophy and the Mirror of Nature..* Oxford: Blackwell.

Rosenfeld, Herbert (1971) 'A Clinical Approach to the Psychoanalytic Theory of the Life and Death Instincts: An Investigation into the Aggressive Aspects of Narcissism', *Int. J. Psycho-anal.* 52: 169-78; reprinted in Spillius (1988), vol. 1, pp. 239-55.

Rudnytsky, Peter L. (1987) *Freud and Oedipus*. N. Y.: Columbia.

Rustin, Margaret (1989) 'Identity: Fragmentation and Recovery in Psychoanalytic Psychotherapy'. *Discourse Social/Social Discourse* 2: 311-19.

Sandberg, Carl (1925) *Abraham Lincoln: The Prairie Years - II*. N. Y.: Scribner's, The Sagamon Edition, 1926.

Sanders, Ed (1972) *The Family: The Story of Charles Manson's Dune Buggy Attack Battalion*. Rupert Hart-Davis; reprinted Panther.

Sandler, Joseph (1987) *From Safety to Superego: Selected Papers*. Karnac Books.

Sandler, Joseph and Sandler, Anne-Marie (1978) 'On the Development of Object Relations and Affects', *Int. J. Psycho-Anal. 59: 285-96.*

Schulz, C. M. (1959) *Peanuts Revisited - Favorites, Old and New*

Searles, Harold F. (1960) *The Nonhuman Environment: In Normal Development and in Schizophrenia.* Madison, CT: International Universities Press.

Sharpe, Ella (1930) 'The Technique of Psychoanalysis'. *Int. J. Psycho-Anal.* 2: 361-86.

Sherwood, Rae (1980) *The Psychodynamics of Race: Vicious and Benign Spirals.* Brighton: Harvester.

Steiner, John (1987) 'The Interplay between Pathological Organizations and the Paranoid-Schizoid and Depressive Positions', *Int. J. Psycho-Anal.* 68: 69-80; reprinted in Spillius, ed. (1988), vol. 1, pp. 324-42.

Stern, A. (1924) 'On the Countertransference in Psychoanalysis'. *Psychoanal. Rev.* 2: 166-74.

Strachey, James (1934) 'The Nature of the Therapeutic Action of Psychoanalysis'. *Int. J. Psycho-Anal.* 15: 127-59.

Strachey. Lytton (1918) *Eminent Victorians;* reprinted Collins, 1959.

Sulloway, Frank J. (1979) *Freud, Biologist of the Mind: Beyond the Psychoanalytic Legend.* Burnett Books/André Deutsch.

Taylor, Charles (1964) *The Explanation of Behaviour.* Routledge & Kegan Paul.

Taylor, Lonn (1983) 'The Open-Range Cowboy of the Nineteenth Century', in Lonn Taylor and Ingrid Marr, *The American Cowboy.* Harper and Row, pp., 16-27.

Theory, Culture and Society (1988) *Postmodernism.* Special Issue, vol. 5, numbers 2-3.

Thom, Martin (1978) 'Anti-racism - Infections of Language', *Wedge* no. 3 (winter), 14-22.

Torres de Beà, E. (1989) 'Projective Identification and Differentiation', *Int. J. Psycho-Anal.* 70:265-74.

Turquet, Pierre (1975) 'Threats to Identity in the Large Group', in L. Kreeger, ed. (1974), pp. 87-144.

Tustin, Frances (1986) *Autistic Barriers in Neurotic Patients.* Karnac.

Tyson, Phyllis and Tyson, Robert L. (1990) *Psychoanalytic Theories of Development: An Integration.* Yale.

Warren, Howard C. (1921) *A History of the Association Psychology.* Constable.

Wiener, Norbert (1950) *The Human Use of Human Beings: Cybernetics and Society.* N. Y.: Houghton Mifflin; reprinted Free Association Books, 1989.

Wiener, Philip. P., ed. (1968-74) *Dictionary of the History of Ideas.* N. Y.: Scribner's, 8 vols.

Winnicott, Donald W. (1947) 'Hate in the Countertransference', in Winnicott (1975), pp. 194-203.

Wright, Peter (1987) *Spy Catcher: The Candid Autobiography of a Senior Intelligence Officer.* N. Y.: Viking.

Glossary

Abnormal A term applied to behaviour or people who have been classed as not normal. A potentially controversial label because of problems in defining *normality*. Abnormality can be defined in several different ways: (1) as behaviour which is different from the *norm* (i.e. unusual); (2) as behaviour which does not conform to social demands; (3) as statistically uncommon behaviour, based on the assumptions of the *normal distribution;* (4) as behaviour which is maladaptive or painful for the individual; or (5) as the failure to achieve self-actualization, the humanistic view. These criteria bring their own problems because they lead to the classification of highly-regarded individuals like artists and social reformers as 'abnormal'.

Abstract thought Thought which uses concepts which do not have an immediate material correspondence, such as justice or freedom. In Piaget's theory of cognitive development, the capacity for abstract thought is only acquired after the age of about 12 years. It is an essential aspect of Piaget's *formal operations* stage.

Achievement The successful reaching of a goal. Used particularly to refer to real-life successes and when evaluating a person's life.

Adolescence The developmental period between childhood and adulthood. In some cultures the transition is very brief and achieved through some form of *rite of passage* but in Western culture it extends from the onset of *puberty* around 12 years of age, to about 17 or 18. Research on adolesence has tended to emphasize the four developmental areas of competence, *individuation, identity* and *self-esteem.*

Aggression A term used in several ways, commonly to describe a deliberate attempt to harm another being. There is no agreed definition, partly because the term is sometimes applied to behaviour (hitting), sometimes to an emotional state (feeling aggressive), and sometimes to an intention (wanting to harm). There are several classifications of different kinds of aggression, the most useful distinction being between *instrumental aggression:* an aggressive act performed in order to achieve some other objective, and *hostile aggression:* motivated by antagonistic feelings and emotions.

Amnesia Loss of memory, normally from physical causes. Retrograde amnesia refers to loss of memory for events prior to the damaging event or disease: loss of memory of the few minutes leading up to severe concussion is the most common example. Anterograde amnesia refers to the loss of subsequent memory: for instance, impairment of the ability to code new memories after brain surgery, or, as found in *Korsakoff's syndrome,* through long-term alcoholism.

Anxiety disorder General term for psychological disorders in which chronic anxiety, with debilitating consequences, is a prominent feature. Includes *panic attacks* and *phobias.*

Astigmatism A disorder of vision in which lines at certain angles are not perceived with the same *acuity* as lines of different orientations. Recent research suggests that astigmatism may arise from the irregular development of *simple* or *complex cells* in the *lateral geniculate nuclei* of the *thalamus* - involved in the primary decoding of visual information.

Autism (i) Thought and fantasy determined entirely by the person's needs and wishes and not constrained by reality in any way. Daydreams are autistic, but the term is usually reserved for the more extreme and permanent removal from reality of *schizophrenic* thought.

(ii) A serious disorder appearing towards the end of infancy, in which the child withdraws from all social contact, which seems to be aversive and distressing. Activity is directed towards inanimate objects and may give evidence of quite high intelligence, but speech is usually minimal. Although it is often called infantile autism, or childhood autism, the condition can persist throughout the person's life. There is little agreement about cause, although a majority of those who work in the area probably believe in an organic predisposition, and even less agreement about treatment.

Aversion therapy A technique of behaviour therapy which involves utilizing the framework of classical conditioning to develop alternative behaviour patterns in the individual. It is done by the association of unpleasant stimuli or consequences with the maladaptive behaviour, such that the behaviour comes to be avoided.

Battered baby A term coined by C. Henry Kempe in 1962 in a paper which first alerted the medical profession to the widespread existence of infants who had been injured by their parents.

Behaviour disorder A general term used to cover a wide range of psychological disorders in which the behaviour of the person is the major concern. More specifically it applies to conditions such as *psychopathy, addictions, and hyperactivity*. One feature of behaviour disorders is that they usually involve symptoms which are likely to bring the sufferer into conflict with society.

Behaviour therapy The process of treating abnormal behaviour by using conditioning techniques to modify maladaptive symptoms. Behaviour therapy includes techniques such as *aversion therapy, systematic desensitization*, and *implosion therapy*.

Biogenic A term applied to behaviours or characteristics with a biological origin.

Bisexual A person whose sexual preference includes people of the same sex as well as those of the opposite sex.

Borderline disorder A disorder of personality. The term was originally applied to people judged to be on the borderline between *neurosis* and *psychosis*, particularly those believed to have an underlying psychotic disorder but who were coping reasonably well. It is now used much more broadly for people with instability in their emotions and interpersonal relationships but whose symptoms do not fit any diagnostic system.

Case history A detailed account of the background and previous experience of a single patient or client, which may be important in therapy or in the understanding of a particular psychological phenomenon, such as anterograde amnesia.

Case study A psychological study involving the detailed investigation of just one particular case, or individual. Case studies are extremely important in many areas of psychology, as they allow for an in-depth analysis of unusual circumstances and their outcomes, which in turn may throw light on more usual psychological events (e.g. the outcome of localized brain damage may serve to highlight the functions of a particular area of the brain). They are also used in situations where a detailed account rather than a limited set of standardized measures are required. However the method has its own difficulties, like subjective decisions about which aspects to describe and difficulties of *replication*.

Castration threat anxiety A Freudian concept, referring to the anxiety experienced by the young boy during the *Oedipus complex*. As the young boy's sexual interest is directed towards his mother, and his father is perceived as a rival for the mother's love, the child develops a fear that the father (being bigger and more powerful than he) may deal with the competition by castrating him.

Catharsis The sudden release of tension or anxiety resulting from the process of uncovering repressed trauma or ideas during psychoanalysis. In a wider context, the process of catharsis is seen as the satisfying release of built-up emotional energy, often through *displacement*, e.g. enthusiastic support of team sports.

Cathexis A term used in *psychoanalytic theory* to refer to the investment of intense energy, desire, or meaning in a person, object or event. In many ways cathexis can be thought of as being the opposite of *catharsis*.

Chemotherapy The treatment of a disorder or clinical problem by means of drugs. Chemotherapy became a popular method of treatment for psychiatric disturbances during the 1950s, when psychoactive drugs such as *chlorpromazine* (largactil) and diazepam (valium) were introduced. The stronger drugs allowed the treatment of persons with extreme behavioural disorders to proceed without physical restraint, and as such became widely used very quickly. In modern days the spectrum of psychoactive drugs available is extremely wide, including such groups as *antidepressants, antianxiety drugs, tranquillizers, amphetamines, barbiturates,* and several more. There is considerable debate as to the ethics and usefulness of many forms of chemotherapy for psychiatric or psychological disorder.

Chronic Continuing over a period of time. The term is usually applied to illnesses to distinguish persisting conditions (such as a depression which has been going on for years) from those that are expected not to last, or at least that have only just started and had a sudden onset. These conditions are called acute.

Cognition A general term used to refer to the 'higher' mental processes. Cognition would generally be taken to include such kinds of mental activity as thinking and conceptualization; *memory, representation,* and mental *imagery; perception* and *attention;* reasoning and decision-making.

Compulsion A repetitive, stereotyped behaviour which is both unnecessary and unwanted but which the individual still feels they have to carry out. Usually associated with obsessions.

Conscience An acquired mental framework for making judgements about the moral 'rightness' or 'wrongness' of actions. The idea of conscience contains strong overtones of duty and obligation. It causes internal anxiety or distress to do things which conflict with the consci

Counselling The term has two rather opposed meanings, (i) Counselling is a form of therapy derived from the *non-directive counselling* of Carl Rogers in which the client is supported while they gain insight into their problem and work on finding their own solution. Within this use, people who offer therapy but who have no formal qualification or whose therapy is carried out as part of another job (e.g. priests), usually call themselves counsellors, (ii) Counselling is also guidance on practical personal problems such as vocational choices, problems in studying etc. These counsellors are much more active in providing information, offering advice etc. In North America this kind of work is an established career and the practitioners are called counselling psychologists.

Daydreaming The activity of engaging in fantasies or imaginative speculations during quiescent waking periods. Some research suggests that daydreaming may be instrumental in promoting positive mental health for the individual, perhaps through the clarification of goals and ambitions.

Dementia A state in which the cognitive abilities of a person are so damaged that they are no longer able to function independently. The term is now used almost exclusively for permanent physical deterioration of the brain. The most common form is senile dementia, which occurs in old age but has a variety of causes.

Depression A reduced state of both physiological and mental functioning, usually associated with feelings of unhappiness. The most common symptoms are a loss of interest and inability to enjoy any experiences, sadness, loss of appetite, sleep disturbances (especially in the morning), passivity, and suicidal thoughts or intentions. However even very severe depressions may only involve a few of these symptoms. The term is used for a very wide range of conditions extending from 'ordinary unhappiness' through to psychotic disorders. Psychologists will therefore indicate when they are using the term to refer to a serious clinical condition either by the context or by attaching further labels: either 'clinical depression' or a specific term for a particular form of depression. The more common of these are: *bipolar depression, endogenous depression* (caused internally), exogenous or *reactive depression*, and *psychotic depression*. Other forms of depression are 'agitated depression' in which the individual is agitated, restless and irritable, and 'retarded depression' when they are slow, apathetic and difficult to get moving.

Displaced aggression Aggressive behaviour which is directed towards a target which is not the original source of frustration. Typically, aggression becomes displaced because the original target is unreachable, or because it would be inexpedient for the individual to direct aggression towards the original. For instance, it may be dangerous for someone to express directly the aggressive feelings generated by an unpleasant boss, and such feelings may become displaced onto family members instead.

Down's syndrome A congenital disorder in which the individual possesses an extra chromosome, giving rise to a series of distinctive physiological characteristics, often accompanied by *mental retardation* and language difficulty. Also called mongolism, a term which originated because of a slight resemblance of children with Down's syndrome to Mongolians, and is now no longer used in the psychological literature.

Ego In Freudian theory, that part of the personality structure that deals with external reality and controls the energies of the *id.* Literally the word means ' I ' and its more general use is to refer to the sense of *identity* or *self.*

Emotional disorder A set of disorders in which children show high levels of *shyness, anxiety,* and *dependency.* The term is also used more broadly to refer to a wide range of psychological disturbances which involve inappropriate emotional experiences, such as *mania and depression.* For this sense an alternative term is *affective disorder.*

Epilepsy A physiological disorder which involves a rapid and unpredicted electrical discharge, starting in the left temporal lobe of the brain and spreading across the cortex. Such a discharge produces temporary changes in mental state, uncontrollable muscular spasms (a fit, or seizure), and leaves the individual with temporary *amnesia* and often feeling very tired. There are many degrees of epilepsy, and although a few unfortunate individuals experience *grand-mal* attacks, which involve a temporary loss of muscular co-ordination and prolonged trembling, many epileptics show little outward sign of the attack. Epilepsy has historically been regarded with a high degree of superstition, but, apart from practical difficulties of lifestyle encountered by epileptics, does not affect the person between attacks. It is difficult to suppress, and anti-epilepsy drugs tend to have strong and unwanted side-effects. In the most severe cases, *split-brain surgery* has been attempted with some degree of success.

Excitation The process by which a *neurone* is rendered likely to fire. Excitation of neural impulses occurs either through direct stimulation of sensory neurones from sense receptors receiving information from the environment, or through the stimulation of a number of *excitatory synapses* making connections with that particular neurone.

Forgetting Broadly speaking, theories of forgetting can be sorted into seven major approaches: decay theory (the idea that memory traces gradually decay over time, unless strengthened by being retrieved); *interference* theory; *amnesia* brought about through physical causes; *motivated forgetting;* lack of appropriate *cues* for retrieval; lack of the relevant context for retrieval; and inadequate processing during storage.

Frustration-aggression hypothesis The proposal, particularly associated with Leon Berkowitz, that aggression is always caused by some kind of frustration. It also tends to be assumed that frustration always leads to aggression. This theoretical model has achieved widespread popularity, and is supported by *comparative* studies of overcrowding in animals as well as by studies of human behaviour.

Group therapy *Psychotherapy* carried out with a number of people, who come together at agreed intervals for the purposes of the therapy. There are many different forms of group therapy, corresponding to most of the varieties of individual therapy, but all could be claimed to have two major advantages over individual therapy. First, cost effectiveness, as a single therapist sees several patients simultaneously. Second, group processes ensure that the participants will have genuine interactions with each other and real emotional experiences which will relate meaningfully to their experiences in daily life, and which can be used effectively by the group therapist.

Hallucination A vivid and convincing mental image which may appear in any sensory modality. The person experiencing it may be unable to believe that no sensory stimulation was involved. Hallucinations are taken as one of the most reliable signs of *schizophrenia* though they may be caused as a side effect of *psychoactive drugs*.

Heuristic Problem-solving strategies which involve taking the most probable or likely options from a possible set, rather than working systematically through all possible alternatives. Heuristics provide a way of reducing a complex problem to a manageable set of tasks with only a slight risk that the solution lies among the alternatives excluded at the start. Heuristics differ from *algorithms* in that they do not guarantee a solution.

Instrumental aggression *Aggression* which occurs because it will result, directly or indirectly, in a desired outcome for the individual showing the aggression.

Intelligence In general, the ability of an individual to understand the world and work out appropriate courses of action. Within psychology there is no more precise definition that is generally accepted, though the old claim that 'intelligence is what *intelligence tests* measure' is uncomfortably acute.

Introvert An individual inclined towards a solitary, reflective lifestyle Introversion is a personality dimension regarded as the opposite of *extraversion*. It was proposed by Carl Jung and incorporated into the *Eysenck Personality Inventory*. Eysenck sees introversion as rising from a higher level of cortical arousal resulting in a lower level of inhibition to the same stimulus, introverted individuals, he argues, do not get bored as easily as extraverts. and so are better at tasks requiring sustained attention or which involve relatively little change in stimulation.

Jet lag A syndrome in which the individual's *circadian rhythms* become out of phase with the surrounding environment, as a result of the rapid crossing of time zones during long-distance travel. This produces feelings of extreme fatigue, and in some cases disorientation, sometimes lasting for several days until the individual adjusts fully to a new time system.

Juvenile delinquent A young person who has been convicted of a criminal offence.

Lesbian A female person who is sexually attracted to members of her own sex.

Lesion A term used to refer to damage to organic tissue which is usually used by psychologists to refer to brain or neural injury. Lesions may be surgical or accidental and may take the form of cutting of specific fibres or pathways. or, of general damage caused, say, by the impact of a heavy object.

Long-term memory (LTM) A term used to describe memories other than those which remain for a few seconds only. According to the *two-process theory* of memory, any information which is retained for any length of time above a few seconds is deemed to have been stored in long-term memory; while that which lasts just for a brief interval (such as a telephone number which has just been looked up) is considered to have been stored in *short-term memory*. Many modern researchers question this commonly accepted distinction, arguing that it is unnecessary and that it fails to discriminate between information retained for varying periods of time. One alternative to this approach has been the *levels of processing* theory, which argues that the decisive factor in how long information is retained is how deeply it has been organized and processed and that there is no need to postulate separate memory stores.

Mania An emotional disorder during which there is elation, talkativeness, impatience with others, over-confidence and an uncontrolled flight of ideas.

Memory The general term given to the storage and subsequent retrieval of information. Memory has been intensively studied by psychologists throughout the history of psychology, and consequently involves an extensive range of theoretical approaches and fields of enquiry. These include the study of episodic memory, everyday memory, *levels of processing*, *encoding* and *representation*, and physiological correlates of memory.

Mental handicap A general term for people of limited intelligence as measured by intelligence tests. The classification of people in these terms raises many difficulties as it labels them in terms of a particular aspect of human ability. Worse, it is an aspect which is highly valued in this culture, and it is measured by tests which many regard as unsatisfactory. In particular, *intelligence tests* are usually standardized on the 'normal' population and they may have less *validity* when applied to other groups. However, people who are mentally handicapped need to be identified so that they can be provided with special resources at an appropriate level and at present, intelligence testing is the most reliable and accurate way of achieving this. The term 'mental handicap' is one in a long line of *labels* which may have been scientifically neutral when first used but which tend to become unacceptable as they pass into the general language as terms of abuse. For example, an earlier grading of mentally handicapped people was as idiots, imbeciles, and morons. The term 'mental deficiency' is sometimes used, particularly for mental handicap which is believed to be due to brain damage. The term's current unpopularity is in part due to a recognition that it is not very productive to attempt to distinguish between organic and non-organic cases. 'Mental retardation' is also widely used, particularly in the American literature.

Mental retardation A general term for limited intelligence. The term tends to carry a misleading assumption that the low intelligence is due to either a slowness of mental functioning, or slow intellectual development.

Multiple sclerosis (MS) A progressive degenerating illness which results in the person gradually losing motor co-ordination and control. MS is produced by the destruction or degeneration of the *myelin sheaths* covering the axons of nerve cells in many parts of the brain, thus slowing down the transmission of information from one part of the brain to another. The process by which this happens is not yet fully understood.

Narcissism A love of the self. The more puritanical approaches to therapy regard narcissism as always undesirable, and when most of a person's affections are fixated upon themself this must be so. However there is plenty of evidence that a healthy degree of affection for the self is essential to maintain *self esteem* and productive functioning.

Narcolepsy A condition in which the person is subjected to sudden, short, uncontrollable episodes of deep sleep. It is much more extreme than the tendency to sleep during psychology lectures and also much rarer.

Nervous breakdown A non-technical term for a more-or-less complete loss of ability to cope with day to day living, showing itself in changes from the person's normal behaviour, such as extreme weepiness or anxiety, and general loss of psychological well-being.

Normality A state which is usually considered to be unremarkable: the opposite *of abnormal.* In attempting to identify normal and abnormal behaviour for the purposes of psychological classification, three alternative approaches are often specified. Firstly, normality is taken to be behaviour which is accepted as usual, or as frequently occurring. Abnormal behaviour is then regarded as behaviour which is uncommon, or at least which is infrequently acknowledged. (In some cases, such as the imagined 'seeing' of a recently dead relative, the experience may actually be very common though not often openly acknowledged). A second definition of normal behaviour, is behaviour which conforms to accepted norms, or social demands. In this event, social consensus becomes a major factor in decisions concerning normality and abnormality. The third approach concentrates on statistically common behaviour, irrespective of consensus. This approach rests on the assumptions of the Gaussian *(normal) distribution*. The problem here is that with this approach, people who are statistically uncommon in a highly valued direction (e.g. of extremely high IQ) are also defined as abnormal.

Obsessive-compulsive disorder A neurotic disorder in which the person is unable to resist spending a lot of time in *obsessional* thoughts which are usually absurd and obscene and carrying out pointless rituals - *compulsions*. The condition is extremely distressing and associated with a high level of anxiety. Psychoanalysis regards it as a personality disorder in which tremendous efforts have been made to suppress and control emotions, with the obsessions and compulsions being the denied aspects of the self which are breaking through the defence;. At an extreme the person may spend so much time on the ritual thoughts and acts that they are unable to do anything else at all. Behavioural approaches view this as an outcome of conditioning processes in which the ritual is reinforced because it provides temporary relief from the anxiety of tackling some real task.

Oedipus complex In Freudian theory, a process occurring during the *phallic stage* (around 3 to 5 years) in which the child wishes to possess the parent of the opposite sex and so sees the same-sex parent as a rival. As this parent is also powerful and successful, the child will feel threatened, but also tends to resolve the conflict by *identifying* with the rival parent. Neo-Freudians, particularly of the *object relations* school, have shifted the emphasis onto earlier relationships with the mother, so that oedipal conflicts have come to be seen either as occurring at a younger age, or as less important as a source of psychological disturbance. The oedipal process is regarded as applying just as much to girls as to boys.

Operant Any unit of behaviour which has an effect (of any kind) on the environment. Also known as operant behaviour, it is the basis of the conditioning of voluntary behaviour. Unless behaviour which has some kind of effect in the environment is produced spontaneously, the *law of effect* cannot come into play, and the behaviour will continue to be emitted more or less randomly.

Panic attack An *anxiety* disorder in which the person experiences sudden and unpredictable attacks of acute anxiety or terror which have no organic cause nor are they a response to any threat in the environment. The anxiety is increased by the fact that the person does not know when another attack will happen, and cannot make any sense out of what is happening to them.

Paranoia A disorder in which the person is dominated by thoughts of persecution, grandeur, and sometimes jealousy. Intellectual functioning is not impaired and great ingenuity may be shown in interpreting every event to fit with the paranoid belief.

Paranoid schizophrenia A *schizophrenic* condition of which the main feature is paranoia, but the consistency of the beliefs found in paranoia is missing.

Personality disorder A term for the very broad class of psychological disorders which seem to arise from long-term characteristics of the person. Roughly, the term applies to conditions which reflect what the person is, rather than how they behave *(behaviour disorders)*. Examples include *psychopathy*, and *paranoia*.

Phobia A *neurotic* disorder in which there is a strong and persistent fear of objects or situations which is not justified by any danger that they pose. The sufferer will be aware that the fear is irrational but will make strenuous attempts to avoid the feared situation. Often, the symptoms can best be seen as attempts to avoid the (very unpleasant) sensations of anxiety, rather than being closely tied to the feared object. Phobias may be attached to a wide range of situations, and particular forms are indicated by putting the appropriate term (usually in Latin or Greek form) in front of the word, as in *agoraphobia* and *claustrophobia*. Specific phobias can usually be treated effectively by behaviour *therapy*, but many, like agoraphobia, incorporate a fear of social interaction, and are more difficult to treat.

Phobic disorder The standard term to cover all of the *phobias*.

Post-hypnotic amnesia The forgetting of information as a result of a suggestion made while the subject was under *hypnosis*, and which occurs after the hypnotic state has finished. Post-hypnotic amnesia is often described by subjects as feeling like 'tip-of-the-tongue' forgetting and can often last for several days.

Post-traumatic amnesia *Amnesia* which results from some kind of accident, such as that resulting from a blow to the head or from severe brain damage.

Psychiatry The medical treatment of abnormal behaviour, or of mental disturbance. Psychiatrists are always medically qualified and therefore, unlike clinical psychologists, may prescribe drugs. Approaches used by psychiatrists range from a concentration on physical methods of treatment through to *psychotherapeutic* approaches in which they may work in very similar ways to some clinical psychologists. Within the National Health Service psychiatrists have a statutory responsibility to deal with all of the cases sent to them. Psychologists do not have this requirement and may therefore be able to spend more time on fewer patients.

Psychosis A term to cover the most severe mental disorders such as *schizophrenia, bipolar disorder,* and *paranoid* *psychosis.* The person in a psychotic state loses contact with reality, has severe disturbances of thought and emotion which are not open to being changed by contrary evidence, and has little or no insight into their condition. Compare *neurosis.*

Psychotherapy Usually the term covers the whole range of psychologically based treatments by which trained practitioners help people who have psychological problems. Sometimes the term is used in a more restricted way, most usually to refer to forms of treatment in which a psychotherapist and a single client tackle the client's problems through talking. Specific forms of psychotherapy may be identified by additional terms, for example *psychodynamics* psychotherapy covers forms of psychotherapy which have been based on one of the psychodynamic theories. Other forms are *non-directive therapy, cognitive psychotherapy* and *rational-emotive therapy.*

Repression A *defence mechanism* by which unacceptable thoughts or desires are forced into the *unconscious.* As with all defence mechanisms, the psychological relief is paid for by having to distort one's perception of reality.

Retrograde amnesia The form of *amnesia* (memory disorder) where the person is unable to remember things which happened before the event which rendered them amnesiac. Retrograde amnes is usually occurs after some form of brain damage, but can happen in a minor way after concussion. It is not uncommon for people who have been in an accident involving severe concussion to lose all memory of the few minutes leading up to the accident.

Role behaviour Behaviour which is considered to be appropriate for someone who is playing a specific social role. For instance, someone playing the role of a shop assistant is expected to behave in certain ways, to be smart, and alert, and to demonstrate specific behaviours such as asking if a customer needs to be served or requires information about prices, etc. Other kinds of behaviour of which the person may be equally capable, such as ballroom dancing, are completely inappropriate to the social role of shop assistant.

Sadism A psychosexual disorder in which a person obtains sexual arousal by inflicting pain or humiliation on another person.

Schizophrenia A broad group *of psychoses* in which emotion is blunted or is not coordinated with thought and behaviour, and in which thought appears to be disordered. Typical symptoms of schizophrenia are *hallucinations*, incoherent speech and thought, and *delusions*. While suffering from schizophrenia a person is unlikely to maintain social relationships or to look after themselves adequately. There is considerable controversy over whether schizophrenia is an *organic* disorder, or whether it happens as a result of life experiences, particularly growing up in certain kinds of family. One of the reasons why this dispute has not been resolved is that there is no very clear and widely accepted definition of schizophrenia, and diagnosis of the condition varies widely in different countries.

Self-consciousness An exaggerated awareness of one's own behaviour, feelings and appearance, combined with a belief that other people are equally aware, interested, and critical. Self-consciousness is often particularly extreme during adolescence.

Senile dementia A loss of intellectual capacity which occurs apparently through a deterioration of the brain. The deterioration may not be directly attributable to ageing, and is often due to degenerative conditions such as Alzheimer's disease, which can also affect younger people.

Spastic Affected by muscular spasms. The term has been used to refer to people suffering from *cerebral palsy* but as it has entered the common language as a derogatory label for clumsiness it is rarely used within psychology.

Special child A term adopted to refer to all children whose qualities or abilities are well outside the normal range. It represents an attempt to avoid the automatically negative implications of terms like *mentally handicapped* and retarded, and to make an association between children who need special resources because of some disadvantage and those who need special attention because they are exceptionally gifted in some way. More recently, the expression 'children with special needs' has been adopted to reduce the possibility of *labelling*.

Stress Usually, the effect on a person of being subjected to noxious stimulation, or the threat of such stimulation, particularly when they are unable to avoid or terminate the condition. Major changes in one's life *(life events)* have been found to be a common source of stress which leave people vulnerable to *depression*. Hans Selye has found similar physiological and psychological reactions to prolonged stress regardless of the nature of the source (see *general adaptation syndrome)*. While stress is unpleasant and often damaging it is also recognized that it may be actively sought (as when apparently sane people jump out of airplanes for fun), and is an important source of motivation. The term is also sometimes used for the source of the stress (noise, poor housing, etc.) but it would be better if such conditions were always called 'stressors'.

Superego In Freudian theory, the third component of personality which forms after the *id* and *ego* have become established. The superego is formed in early childhood by internalizing the parents' system of rewards and punishments, so that the child comes to operate according to these rules even when the parents are not present. It is not quite the same thing as the conscience as it retains an infantile version of the parents' rules which is likely to be severe and intolerant. The adult conscience may be much more realistic and sophisticated and so may come into conflict with the superego.

Syndrome A set of symptoms or events which tend to occur together functionally.

Telepathy The communication of *cognitions* (thoughts, etc.) by other means than those understood in conventional science. There is considerable dispute over whether the phenomenon occurs, and its definition precludes rational explanation: if a communication can be explained, it is not telepathy.

Temperament The stable aspects of the character of an individual, which are often regarded as biologically rooted, and as providing the fundamental dispositions which, through interaction with the environment, produce the *personality*.

Therapy The treatment of an individual by physical or psychological means. When applied to psychological treatments, the term implies that the client is ill and should be cured.

Transcendental meditation A technique derived from Hindu practice, of sustained concentration on a brief phrase *(mantra)* to induce *relaxation*.

Transsexual A person who changes sex, either from male to female or from female to male, usually through a course of hormone therapy and surgery. Although typically transsexuals have always experienced themselves as being 'really' the other sex, the main part of transsexualism involves the learning of a new sex role. Many transsexuals have to spend an extensive period of time, at least a couple of years, passing as a member of their desired sex before being allowed treatment.

Unconscious A lack of *conscious* awareness. The most important use of the term is in psychoanalytic theory as a reference to mental activity which is not available to consciousness because it concerns material which is too threatening to the *ego* to be recognized directly. Freud believed that the unconscious has its own way of working which is different from that of the conscious mind. For example there is no awareness of time in the unconscious so all threats are felt as if they were still present, even if the source of the threat disappeared years ago.

Unipolar depression A depression which is similar in form to a *bipolar disorder* but in which the manic phase is absent; the person simply has the depressive periods without the swings to mania.

Verbal memory This term is used in two main ways. Firstly to mean the storing of mental images by using words as a form of coding for information. In this case, verbal memory is simply meant as a variation of *symbolic representation*, with all the associated features and advantages. Secondly, the term is used to mean memory for words. Much laboratory research on memory, especially in the early years, concentrated initially on asking subjects to memorize lists of words, partly because subjects were able to state clearly exactly what they remembered, which was not always easy with visual or auditory images. But there is considerable recent evidence to suggest that this form of learning is qualitatively different from the way that people remember connected prose or speech, and even more different from everyday memory. In its most general sense, verbal memory includes memory for speech and prose.

Voluntary behaviour Behaviour which forms a deliberate action on the part of the individual. Such behaviour is usually contrasted with *involuntary*, or *reflexive*, behaviour. *Operant conditioning* and the higher forms of learning are usually concerned with the training of voluntary behaviour except in the case of *biofeedback'*, *classical* *conditioning* is typically concerned with involuntary behaviour.

Withdrawal symptoms Temporary physical disorders which occur as a result of the subject failing to receive their normal dose of a drug on which they have become *dependent*. Withdrawal symptoms can be quite severe, depending both on the drug concerned and on the extent to which the subject has become *habituated to* the drug. Many ordinary drugs, such as caffeine, can produce quite strong withdrawal symptoms if the individual has previously had a high regular intake and suddenly ceases to take the drug altogether. The existence or otherwise of withdrawal symptoms is one of the main indicators of physiological *addiction*.

Xenophobia An irrational and excessive fear of strangers or strange, (foreign) cultures, which can often become converted into intense, jingoistic patriotism, and/or racial or cultural *prejudice*.

Yavis A term used to describe the typical patient considered suitable for *psychoanalysis*. The term stands for 'young, attractive, verbal, intelligent and successful'. Patients who don't fit these criteria are frequently allocated to other less expensive forms of treatment, e.g. *behaviour therapy*. Although this idea is only semi-serious, it contains more than a grain of truth in terms of the types of patients which many psychoanalysts prefer to treat.

Index